T0234511

Simplicity in Safety Investigations

This innovative book aims to bring the science of safety into a simple and practical approach to investigating workplace incidents. As a basis, it uses the ideas of some of the great safety science thinkers of our time. These include Sidney Dekker, Todd Conklin, Erik Hollnagel, Daniel Kahneman, James Reason and Dylan Evans, alongside others and the author's own extensive industry experience.

Simplicity in Safety Investigations: A Practitioner's Guide to Applying Safety Science will better equip readers to deal with incident investigations by helping them understand the science behind investigation techniques, and by exploring coaching and leadership styles that help them ask better questions both before and after workplace incidents. The first two chapters of the book focus on our mindset as we approach and undertake investigations, and the simple things we all must do before an investigation starts. The third chapter is a step-by-step guide on how to undertake both simple and more detailed workplace incident investigations. Chapter 4 is reserved for a more detailed review and set of explanations around the science and thinking behind the method and approach.

This book serves as an easy-to-follow, real-world reference for supervisors, managers and safety practitioners across many industries.

Ian Long has worked for over twenty years in Health and Safety roles in the minerals extraction and processing industry. As the managing director of his own consultancy business, he now provides in-the-field coaching and coach-the-coach activities with leaders, along with training and facilitation of fatality and other significant incident investigations.

Simplicity in Safety Investigations

A Practitioner's Guide to Applying Safety Science

Ian Long

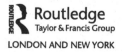
Routledge
Taylor & Francis Group

LONDON AND NEW YORK

First published 2018
by Routledge
2 Park Square, Milton Park, Abingdon, Oxon OX14 4RN

and by Routledge
711 Third Avenue, New York, NY 10017

Routledge is an imprint of the Taylor & Francis Group, an informa business

British Library Cataloguing-in-Publication Data
A catalogue record for this book is available from the British Library

Library of Congress Cataloging-in-Publication Data
Names: Long, Ian, 1961– author.
Title: Simplicity in safety investigations : a practitioner's guide to applying safety science / Ian Long.
Description: First Edition. | New York : Routledge, 2018. |
Includes bibliographical references and index.
Identifiers: LCCN 2017017298 | ISBN 9781138097711 (hardback) |
ISBN 9781138097735 (pbk.) | ISBN 9781315104737 (ebook)
Subjects: LCSH: Industrial safety. | Industrial hygiene.
Classification: LCC HD7261 .L55 2017 | DDC 363.1/065–dc23
LC record available at https://lccn.loc.gov/2017017298

ISBN: 978-1-138-09771-1 (hbk)
ISBN: 978-1-138-09773-5 (pbk)
ISBN: 978-1-315-10473-7 (ebk)

Typeset in Bembo
by Out of House Publishing

Contents

Figures

Preface

You would have thought that after more than a century we would have learned how to investigate industrial incidents and events effectively. Yet many of us still struggle. Why is this, and how can we get better? During this book, we will explore a way of approaching workplace incident investigations that I hope you will find pleasing, simple, modern, and that builds on the shoulders of great thinkers and processes of the past and present.

Over the last century or so the methods for carrying out workplace incident investigations have changed significantly. Many of these changes have been due to evolving views and thoughts on the causes of safety-related incidents and the drivers of human behaviour. We only need to look at the safety handbook given to all employees at the DuPont explosives factory in New Jersey at the start of 1915 to get a sense of where we were and to see what is in many ways the start of the journey we are still on. DuPont said:

> Most accidents, whether incurred at the works or in the home, are due:
>
> To not knowing what is right.
>
> To doing what is known to be wrong.
>
> To not caring whether the act is right or wrong.
>
> To not stopping to think whether it is right or wrong.

In 1915, we can see there was a tendency to believe that the human was the predominant cause of industrial accidents. It was how we viewed the world at the time; that the human factor is one that needs to be controlled and when something goes wrong, it is the human component that failed.

In the same handbook, DuPont explains that 65.1% of the accidents were the fault of a worker and 8.6% were the fault of the employer. It is interesting to note that in the view of DuPont in 1915, 22.9% of accidents were caused by "risk of employment", which was designated under a category named "unavoidable".

So, what has been going on in safety over these last hundred years or so? Both Eric Hollnagel in *Safety I and Safety II* and Sydney Dekker in *Safety Differently* talk about where we have come from in the world of safety, before going on to explore where they feel we ought to go in the future. In essence, the focus of safety and the investigation of safety-related workplace incidents has been, and continues to be, linked to the technology of the time. As Hollnagel states, "When there was no electricity, there could be no short circuits. When there was no radio communications, there could be no transmission errors." As the interactions between people and technology have changed, so have our views regarding the causality and mechanisms of failure in the workplace. As can also been seen in the DuPont example above and in the works of Dekker and Hollnagel, in the early parts of the twentieth century the causes of workplace incidents were very much focussed on the human component of the system. This all changed after the Second World War when it was realized that the way the equipment and the person interacted could have a large impact on safety and the likelihood of mistakes being made. At that point the pendulum swung away from trying to fit the human to the machine and towards understanding the drivers of human behaviour more deeply. This continued throughout the second half of the twentieth century. Investigation methodologies that were developed through the latter part of the century such as ICAM (Incident Cause Analysis Method) relied, and continue to rely heavily on the organizational components of the incident as something to fix rather than focussing on the individual.

Even though it is just over 100 years since DuPont shared its views of incident causation with its employees by way of the safety handbook we talked about earlier, we are still trying to work out what drives, or creates, workplace incidents. Over the past twenty years in particular, significant advances have occurred in the science surrounding safety and human factors. I would say our understanding of human actions, behaviour, and 'human error' has developed in leaps and bounds since I first started doing workplace incident investigations back in the mid-1990s, and has certainly improved exponentially since 1915. It is time to embed our thinking firmly into the twenty-first century. Of course, we should not throw the baby out with the bathwater and so the question that we are attempting to answer here in this book is how do we combine the accumulated body of knowledge on incident investigations, the things that already exist, with the science and ideas of the latest thinkers and practitioners within the worlds of safety and human factors?

This, according to Brynjolfsson and McAfee in *The Second Machine Age* is the definition of innovation: "The true work of innovation is not coming up with something big and new, but instead recombining things that already exist." They go on to describe this particular form of innovation as "recombinant innovation" which I think accurately describes this book. I have taken what I believe to be the best bits of various theories, ideas and practices and recombined them into a workplace incident investigation approach that works, is easy to use and is relevant for the vast majority of workplace incidents we come across. My intention is to help people understand how simple a workplace incident investigation can be. In other words, how do we innovate for the purpose of improving investigations, improving in-the-field leadership conversations and help drive the creation of safe workplaces?

We are attempting to create a way of being in incident investigations that is firmly based in science and also brings in the practical – what works and what doesn't. I want to show how we can better understand the drivers of an incident by simply thinking a little differently about safety, decision-making and leadership. I am a firm believer in the saying "thinking about how we think about safety improves safety". It is for this reason that I focus quite a bit on our approach and mindset as we embark on an investigation. Todd Conklin, in his latest book *Pre-Accident Investigations: Better Questions*, talks about the fact that it is not about 'how' we do investigations, it is about how we 'think' about doing investigations that is important.

I have been working in the field of occupational health and safety for over twenty years now, in roles ranging from safety advisor through to vice president of health and safety and many in between. Now I own my own company, Raeda Consulting, where I continue to help as many people as I can to be the best they can be in the areas of workplace incident investigations, safety leadership and coaching. During these last twenty years or so I have seen and used a number of investigation techniques; ranging from simple tools such as Root Cause Analysis, 5-whys, events and conditions charting, through to MORT (Management Oversight and Risk Tree) analysis, Fishbone (Ishikawa) diagrams, and the more workload-intensive but eminently workable ICAM, included in Appendix B.

This book attempts to share an approach to incident investigations that incorporates some of the old thoughts and ideas with the latest advances in safety science whilst maintaining a firm practical base. The techniques I will describe are elements from the New View, Safety II and Safety Differently styles of thinking and application. The approaches I describe and explore in this book have been proven successful in action and are simple to use.

My intent is not to try to replicate the works of Hollnagel, Dekker or others by spending time exploring the science of the New View or Safety Differently; as I believe the authors do that far more effectively in their books and papers than I ever could. I list many of these in the Bibliography at the end of the book. My aim is to help you understand what is important in investigations, why that is so, and just as importantly, how to practically run workplace incident investigations.

A conversation that pops up often during many of my investigation workshops is around whether an incident investigation attempts to understand the past, or to create the future. To me, incident investigations are all about the future. Yes, we investigate incidents so that we can understand the past, but investigations are primarily about projecting what we learn during the investigation into the future. Investigations are about making changes in the way we do things so that we can create safe work going forward. Investigations are about learning. Todd Conklin goes so far as to not even use the word "investigation" and talks about "learning teams" instead of "investigation teams" in his work. I have also heard and read others who talk about "incident reviews" instead of investigations.

The whole purpose of an incident investigation is to explore the past so that we can build a future. A future where things go right, not a future where things go wrong. Incident investigations are all about learning. Unfortunately, in many of the incident investigations I have seen or reviewed, a lot of focus and energy is consumed in an attempt to find out who did what wrong; and who did something they should not have done. Workplace incident investigations should not be about finding blame, or perceiving someone's actions as 'wrong'. Nor should they be about seeking out who was involved in the incident and then holding them 'accountable' for their choices or their behaviour. Incident investigations are about exploration. They are about discovering the way we do things on a daily basis and finding out what was going on in the mind of those involved in the incident. They are also about exploring ourselves; how we approach the investigation itself, what we bring to the table and what conversations we have with ourselves and with others. Once again, workplace incident investigations are all about learning.

Sydney Dekker sums up how human error plays a part in incident investigations very clearly when he talks about 'human error' as being the start of the investigation conversation – not the end of it. You will notice that throughout the book I do not talk about 'human error' much. Rather, I talk about actions taken by individuals or teams that had unintended outcomes. This is very intentional and Chapter 4 of the book covers some of the theoretical discussions behind this.

Simplicity in Safety Investigations is intended for those of you who want to explore the reasons behind things not quite going according to plan at work. A big bonus, though, is that the concepts, ideas and practices contained in the book can also just as easily be used to explore the reasons behind things going right as they can when exploring the reasons behind things going wrong. We will talk more about this later. Principally the book concerns the fields of occupational safety, health and the environment, but could also be used in the areas of maintenance, operations, construction, process, patient safety or even financial outcomes. For the purposes of simplicity, I will use 'safety' as a surrogate for these other outcomes throughout the book. The concepts and tools described are applicable to any industry; whether that is mining, oil and gas, healthcare, manufacturing, construction or major project management. I was firmly reminded of this during a recent re-read of *Patient Safety* by Sidney Dekker. In the case of healthcare and patient safety, the content and specifics change and the 'safety' is about the patient, the recipient of the work, not just the person doing the work. The philosophy and the tools are happily the same.

A question that may be popping into your head about now is 'Why?' Why do we need another book about investigations? Who is it written for? Why now? What is wrong with the ones we already have? And who does Ian Long think he is to be writing it in the first place? I feel these are all valid questions and will provide some insight into my thoughts on them.

I am convinced that the way forward for safety, including investigations into workplace incidents, the coaching of leaders around safety concepts and even investigations into things that go right, does not lie in the pure application of tools and methods that have been proven to work in the past. The science of safety has moved on, along with the technological changes we see in most other fields. It is time to up the level of effort and work with respect to helping people think about how they think about safety, how we think about workplace incidents and how we work within our workplaces. I feel there is a need to pull together aspects of the past and tie them into the science of the present. Innovation is needed. It is time to bring all aspects together in a simple and practical way that doesn't throw the baby out with the bathwater but does allow the conversation to include concepts and ideas that are being discussed amongst the boffins, mavens and other bright-minded beings. That is why it is time for a book like this. I have reviewed thousands of workplace incident investigations and my feeling is that many of the investigation methods we currently use are simply not accessible to the people most needing them – front-line supervisors, superintendents, technical specialists and professionals. Using a bit of recombinant innovation to explore what has worked well in the past with the latest thinking and safety science has resulted in this book.

Who is this book for? If you are required to run an investigation at your workplace then this book is for you. Its intent is to prompt thinking and offer new ways of looking at old problems, sharing with you ideas and practical ways of carrying out investigations. If you have people reporting to you then this book is for you as I believe that the questions and conversations we have after a workplace incident should be the same as the questions and conversations we have before an incident occurs – during our normal day-to-day leadership activities. If you are a student of safety, human factors, engineering, management or leadership, then this book may also be for you as well. It offers a way of thinking about and exploring your mindset, the conversations you have and the leadership you show after a workplace incident in your business. If you are a safety professional looking for a way of approaching and talking about incident investigations that is a bit different, yet is very practical, you may also find some interesting information within these pages.

What level of investigation should we do?

Many organizations spend excessive time contemplating this question instead of just getting on with the investigation. The secret to knowing what level of investigation you should do after a workplace incident is in having the answer ready before you are asked the question. Think about the question as you prepare your incident investigation protocol or procedure and include guidance on the matter. Don't wait until the incident has occurred to work out your investigation options as this often leads to management teams having panicked conversations that delay the start of the investigation. Keep the decision-making process as simple as possible though. Creating mind-numbing decision matrices and processes will only complicate things and put people off.

Deciding on the level of investigation is not related to the actual outcome of the incident. Rather, it is about the potential consequences. At one end of the spectrum lie those incidents that were never going to be anything other than what they were – with no plausible potential for a fatality or major loss. At the other end lie the "Wow, that was really close. We nearly killed Sally"-type incidents.

Let's take the example of a cut on a knee that required a couple of stitches. In most jurisdictions, this level of injury would be classified as a medical treatment injury and could very well be called a recordable injury in many organizations. The classification should not drive the type of investigation you carry out, however; the potential consequences should. In this example, the depth and complexity of the investigation should match the potential. If the cut was caused by a slip with a screwdriver, then we should choose to complete a simple investigation. If the incident was caused by a truck driving past at 40 kilometres per hour and clipping someone's knee, then we should do a more detailed incident investigation because we could have easily killed the worker. I have attempted to structure the book so that you can vary the level of depth – or complexity – of an investigation within each section depending on your needs, all without changing the underlying processes or science. For the sake of clarity, I will use the term 'Outcome Analysis' for simple investigations. This level of investigation is designed to cover off on the vast majority of workplace incident investigations that you may need to carry out. I will then use the term 'detailed investigations' or sometimes 'more detailed incident investigations' for those special few incidents that could have been really nasty and that often have significant organizational-level components. The term 'Outcome Analysis' comes from the idea that for these low-level investigations, we are analysing the unexpected outcome of work. This could be a positive or a negative outcome.

I was running an investigation facilitation workshop at a plant recently when one of the area managers asked me about an incident they had just had and asked for my thoughts and advice. The incident was this: during a maintenance shutdown that they were in the middle of undertaking, a maintainer was working about 8 metres above the ground installing a valve in a line when he dropped a large spanner and it fell to the ground. Naturally, one of the first questions I was asked was related to what level of investigation should they do. As I mentioned earlier, the answer lies in the potential consequence of the incident, not on what happened in this specific case. There is no doubt that a spanner weighing a couple of kilograms falling about 8 metres has the potential to kill someone if it lands on their head. But was it possible in this particular case? In our conversation, I was told that the manager already knew that the crew had spent some time before they started the job thinking about what could go wrong during their task, and they had identified that an object could fall or be dropped – and if it was heavy, it could kill someone. As a result of this thinking, they had put a barrier in place below their workspace, creating a drop zone so that nobody could find themselves in the line of fire.

The conversation then turned to the definition of the incident. Was it a near miss? Was it a failure? Or was it a success due to the fact that the barrier worked as intended? I have heard Todd Conklin in one of his podcasts talk about the concept of a 'successful failure'. I like that idea. There was a failure inasmuch as the team lost control of a heavy tool a long way above the ground, but there was also a success as the barrier functioned exactly as planned; the spanner fell into the drop zone and there was no possibility of a fatal incident.

So, for this successful failure we should not do a detailed investigation. We talked about this and the manager felt that the maintainer who dropped the spanner should be held accountable for not keeping control of his tools. They ended up doing a low-level Outcome Analysis involving the crew themselves in the investigation process with one of the outcomes being that the team got to tell their story – or their account, if you like – of the incident to other teams as a lesson on the importance of barriers and controls.

Of course there will be grey areas, where it is not always obvious whether it is more appropriate to go with a simple Outcome Analysis or a detailed incident investigation. One way to help you sort through this dilemma is to see how many times you need to add "and if…" to the story before a fatality or major loss becomes truly plausible.

For example, in the earlier case of the knee being clipped by a passing truck; "*And if* the person was one step further out into the road, he could have been struck by the truck and killed". That one "and if" indicates we should carry out a detailed incident investigation. In the case of a person leaning back on a chair, falling over and hitting his head on a wall behind them, you could add "*and if* the wall had not been so close and he fell all the way to the ground, *and if* there had been a 6 inch nail sticking out of the ground, *and if* the position of the nail was such that it hit him at the base of the skull and went into his brain then he could have died" – that is too many "and ifs" and a simple Outcome Analysis will do – if you are going to do any investigation at all, this is it.

Another aspect worth considering is the level of resources you are prepared to invest in the investigation. Investigations take time and require people to run them and participate in them. A simple Outcome Analysis-style investigation may only take three or four people a couple of hours to complete whereas a detailed investigation may tie up five or six people for a week. A manager-level or high-quality superintendent-level person should always be the leader of a detailed investigation, but if you are carrying out five detailed investigations a week, then dedicating a manager-level resource to each of these may not be achievable, or even desirable.

The reason why I strongly support giving a manager-level person the role of incident investigation leader when you are running detailed incident investigations is that they tend to think at a systems level. If the detailed incident investigation is going to fix things at the level of management systems, then you need someone who tends to think at that higher level; at the level of overarching management systems and standards.

It's important to strike the right balance when challenging whether the incident is a truly plausible fatality incident that requires a detailed investigation or not. There can be a tendency for people to want to carry out detailed investigations for all reportable injuries and illnesses. I discourage this. Reserve your powerful, high-horsepower, detailed investigations for those incidents that are truly plausible fatalities. You should absolutely investigate medical treatment injuries and illnesses, restricted work cases and lost time cases – but devote your time and effort to them according to their potential consequences.

Another concept well worth understanding and thinking about as you develop your protocol for determining what level of investigation to undertake is the Efficiency–Thoroughness Trade-Off (ETTO) principle. The ETTO principle is explained by Erik Hollnagel in his book by the same name (*The ETTO Principle – Efficiency–Thoroughness Trade-Off: Why Things that Go Right Sometimes Go Wrong*). Hollnagel explains that we cannot adequately serve both masters of efficiency and thoroughness. There is always a trade-off, hence the name ETTO. I have seen it used as a verb also. To ETTO, or not to ETTO? That is the question. Actually, it is not the right question at all, because we use the ETTO principle each and every time we undertake an incident investigation or make a decision.

In the case of workplace incident investigations, if we have an unlimited budget and all the time in the world, then we can be extremely thorough in our investigation. It might take six or twelve months and a team of fifty to complete. If, on the other hand we are resource-constrained, which is the more likely reality, we may choose a far smaller team and expect delivery of a completed incident investigation report within a few weeks. This is more efficient in terms of minimizing time and dollar spend, but the resultant investigation will not be as thorough. It is always a trade-off.

I was reading the *Columbia Accident Investigation Board* report recently and noted that the investigation into the 2003 Space Shuttle Columbia disaster involved a thirteen-member board, some 120 staff, a review of 30,000 documents and 200 formal interviews. It took seven months to complete. Clearly, the board was able to apply a lot more thoroughness than efficiency in their multiple fatality investigation. Unlike what the majority of us would apply to the sort of workplace incident we may be investigating. The report is a fascinating read, incidentally.

Another problem with doing too many detailed incident investigations is that it can run the risk of devaluing the process. I have seen this with ICAM (described in Appendix B). The investigations can easily become a burden and then a 'tick and flick' activity that really does not help anyone. Reserve your more detailed incident investigations and ICAMs for high-potential incidents, apply the best team you are able to and then give them the time and resources they need to do their job to the best of their ability.

Rather than having two clearly separate investigation processes, I describe methods that can be applied as a continuum going from simple Outcome Analyses at one end all the way through to complicated fatality-level investigations at the other, whilst still using the same underlying technology and science. This allows flexibility. It is important to start out with a clear intent regarding the level of investigation, but we will see that we can make adjustments as we go. I have included a range of options within each step of the process so that you can make the call as to the level of investigation as you progress through it. I have found this works much better in practice than creating some artificial segregation between simple and complex investigation techniques.

We will explore the following in more detail in Chapter 3, but it is worth setting the scene for what the steps are in an investigation. Not all apply in all cases, but generically, a workplace incident investigation has the following steps:

Scene preservation
Interviewing (versus taking statements)
Data- and information-gathering – PEEPO
Determining Work-As-Done, Work-As-Normal and Work-As-Intended
Exploration of the gaps between Work-As-Done, Work-As-Normal and Work-As-Intended
Build the story (Incident Pathway Statement)
SMARTS actions
Reports

For your consideration:

Does your organization have a method or process for deciding what level of workplace incident investigation to carry out?

Are you providing the right level of management involvement in incident investigations?

Ask yourself and your management team why your organization carries out investigations. What are they looking for?

Using this book and the techniques described within it for positive investigations

Just like in the section above, at various points in the book you will see '*For your consideration*' ideas and questions related to the topic being explored. These include ideas that are for you to consider applying not only after an incident during an investigation, but also before an incident in your day-to-day work. This is because I believe that the questions we ask after an incident should be the same as those we ask before an incident. The same science, theories and thoughts lie behind the work we do on a day-to-day basis when things go right as they do in a workplace incident when things have gone wrong. This can be taken a step further in terms of carrying out an investigation on 'positive' incidents as well as for 'negative' incidents. The question we are asking in positive Outcome Analyses is really "How did we get it right?", or "How do we get it right so often?", or even "How are we managing to get this right so much of the time?" We know that workplace incidents are very rare events and yet we tend to focus our resources and efforts on understanding the work only when something goes wrong.

As you read through the various sections of the book as well as the more directive '*For your consideration*' sections, I invite you to think about how you can use the language, mindset, processes and thoughts to aid your understanding of how your business manages to get things right so many times. An example of when to consider how we have got it right is when you have had a good run of safety outcomes, say a large number of days without a recordable injury. In this case, you can do a simple Outcome Analysis investigation in order to understand how you did it. Another example is when you have one area of your business that does things really well, that always looks good, that seems not to have incidents and leaves you with a good feeling when you visit. In this case, you can carry out a simple Outcome Analysis to understand what they are doing differently to others. A third example is when you have one shift doing things much faster or more productively than other shifts, then you can ask some questions and do a simple investigation to get behind it all.

At an investigation facilitator training workshop recently, I asked for a show of hands for people who had crossed a pedestrian crossing in the last two years when the lights were red. I got a 100% show of hands. Everyone in the workshop had broken the law a significant number of times during the last two years by crossing on a red pedestrian light. After berating them for being a room full of criminals, which was fun considering some were senior managers, I asked whether any of them had got hit by a car whilst crossing the road. The answer was a firm "NO". I asked why. I then asked, "How are we managing to get this right so much of the time? How are we crossing the road against the rules so often and not getting hurt?" This is a classic start to a positive investigation. The simple fact is that we are crossing the road many times and not getting hurt, yet not following the rules. Something must be working. Yes, this is partly due to the problem of assuming a good outcome must have come from a good decision and a bad outcome must have come from a bad decision but it is also a reflection that rare events occur rarely, and yet we build confidence when the outcome is OK that we are doing it 'right'. Suffice to say that we did a short 'positive' investigation. We started by asking about the details of how people actually cross the road, how the work is normally being done in other words. We also established what the variability within the team was with respect to road-crossing techniques. In the case of this group, there was a near consistent behaviour of always stopping at the roadside, looking both ways and only crossing if the road was clear in both directions. One person said that she often looked only one way, then crossed halfway, stopped and looked the other way before continuing. Others looked both ways, waited for clear traffic, then crossed halfway and stopped again, checking the traffic before continuing. There was a view that what the team generally did was not always the same as others observed on the pedestrian crossings, with some people attempting to cross lane by lane when each was clear, some always waiting for green and some just walking regardless of the traffic. It was felt that there was a mixture of safe and not so safe methods. Once we had established how the group crossed roads, we looked at the rules. The legislation of the state and government guidance material covered it well and was very specific. We looked at the specific differences between the way the work is done by the team and the government guidance and legislation. There were many elements that were the same, such as stopping and looking both ways. The only major difference was the crossing when the little light was red. We highlighted this aspect and tried to understand what was driving this difference between work as it is done and work as it is intended by the government. It was established that the way the team members did short risk assessments in their minds before crossing the road on a red light was safer than blindly following the rule of being OK to cross when the light was green.

The outcome of the investigation was a decision not to change behaviour but to emphasize within the team the need to always stop and assess a situation before doing anything, regardless of the rule or legislation. In some cases, they felt this was above and beyond the legal requirement and would sometimes yield absolute compliance, and at other times, a deviation from the rule. The team were OK with this approach. I felt this was very mature, although I am not sure they were ready to apply such logic and freedom directly back into their workforces without additional controls such as written risk assessments, Task Hazard Analyses, etc. when the rules are going to be broken or bent.

Some essentials

In order to be able to navigate this book, I feel that we need to explain a few words as they are intended to be used. There are always terms and acronyms that are used in one industry but not in another. I will use the following words and terms quite frequently.

Supervisor: A first-line leader or manager of a small team of 'workers'. The 'workers' could be maintainers or operators in a mine or in a processing plant. They could be professionals such as nurses or engineers. For my purposes, supervisor is synonymous with foreman, leading hand, boss, area coordinator, shift boss or ward-based clinical nurse manager.

Superintendent: The next-up manager above a supervisor. Typically, a superintendent has a number of supervisors reporting to them.

Task Hazard Analysis (THA). This is synonymous with job hazard analysis, job safety analysis, task analysis and job safety and environmental analysis and many other similar tools. A THA is a description of the steps required to undertake a work activity with each step broken down to the hazards and controls associated with each step. It is a tool that is usually created by the team carrying out the work immediately prior to the commencement of that work, although sometimes it is pre-prepared beforehand and then reviewed by the work team prior to the work activity.

Acknowledgements

I often wonder whether authors realize the impact they have on their readers – whether they understand the size and extent of the shadow they cast. This book can be traced back to my reading and thinking about a definition of safety coined by Sidney Dekker. In his words, safety is "the presence of positive capabilities, capacities and competencies that make things go right and not as the absence of things that go wrong".

Contemplating this view changed my views on safety and is a direct cause of my exploration and contemplation of the works of Dekker (specifically *Safety Differently*, *Behind Human Error*, *The Field Guide to Understanding 'Human Error'* and *Just Culture*); Erik Hollnagel (*Safety I and Safety II*, and his excellent works on the notions of resilience and ETTO); Dylan Evans (*Risk Intelligence*); Daniel Kahneman (*Thinking, Fast and Slow*); and Todd Conklin (*Pre-Accident Investigations*, *Better Questions* and his podcast that goes by the name of *The Pre-Accident Investigation Podcast*). What followed was the realization that the way we see safety and how we investigate workplace incidents does not match their world-views. I thank those listed above for this insight. I then felt that I needed to share my thoughts with others. The writing of *Simplicity in Safety Investigations* is the result.

Thanks go to Martin Webb and his team for some great conversations, early trialling and fine-tuning of the methods you see here. A special thanks goes to the support of my family. In particular, my wife Trish, who has encouraged me and pushed me to get this book completed and to Paige, my journalist daughter who – at great personal effort and time expense – improved a lot of my grammar, and also acted as my style guide.

Guy Loft of Routledge has been a fantastic support. His advice and thoughts resulted in a significant structural change and a major rewrite. He has been very supportive of me and the idea of the book throughout its gestation.

Simplicity in Safety Investigations has gone through a number of iterations and changes – many of which were influenced by a band of peers, friends and colleagues. They kindly reviewed early drafts and offered suggestions and improvements as the book slowly moved from idea to reality. These include Karen Ross, Phil Abraham, Jen Jaksic, Chris Long, Tiffany Roxburgh, Mark and Gayle Emmerson. Thanks guys. Many thanks also go to Kelly Steckel of TRE Consultants, who created the great illustrations.

I also thank you for being interested enough to pick up the book and read this far. Hopefully you continue the journey, enjoy it, and get something out of it. I would love to hear your thoughts and questions: ian. long@raeda.com.au.

1   Mindset and approach

What do you want out of an incident investigation? What are you looking for? What is your initial response when you hear about an incident at your workplace? What do you feel in your heart when one of your team tells you that someone has been hurt at your work? Do you want to blame someone or learn something? The answers to some or all of these questions will dictate not only how you are perceived as a leader, but will also have a direct bearing on the quality of any incident investigation that may be done. We all look at things through tinted glasses and listen to things through tinted earplugs. These earplugs and glasses are not always rose-coloured and they can greatly impact how we think about things and how we react to them.

This idea that thinking about how we think about workplace incidents impacts the quality of the resultant investigation has a strong analogy in industrial safety more generally that is worth contemplating. This is the idea that 'thinking about how we think about safety improves safety'. In both the specific case of workplace incident investigation quality and the general case of the improvement in safety, much of it is to do with our mindset as leaders, as practitioners, as operators, technicians or maintainers.

If you want to know what is going on in someone's mind, watch their body language and listen to their speech. What happens in the mind becomes the words used and then the actions taken. It is exactly the same with respect to our bodies and speech when we are confronted with a workplace safety incident. Our bodies and speech will give away our thoughts on the subject. When we hear about an incident our reactions will reflect our state of mind at the time. The same thing happens during the interview phase of an investigation. What we think we are looking for and how we choose to focus our mind will greatly influence the investigation's direction and the outcomes we experience.

This idea of What-You-Look-For-Is-What-You-Find is just as true for simple incident investigations as it is for large-scale and complex incident investigations.

For example, if we approach an investigation with a view that we are owed information, that there is an individual at fault somewhere and that it is the investigation team's job to find out what someone did and why, then we will find that person and we will most likely be perceived as accusatory and supportive of a blame culture.

The phrasing of the questions we ask – in addition to our body language as we ask those questions – will reveal our biased viewpoint and our way of thinking. The game will also be given away during the conversations we have within the investigation team and in the report we write.

So, if we set ourselves up to be inquisitive, to seek answers and to understand what was going on in the minds of those closest to the incident, we will tend to come across as genuinely interested and caring. We can then gather a great deal more information and gain a much better understanding of what went on and why.

The idea of having a clear and purposeful mindset during an investigation is very similar to the mindset we seek within leadership. In many ways leadership is about raising or maintaining performance through conversation and action. And the degree of authenticity and situational self-awareness we have will affect our leadership. This also applies to our mindset and thus to our leadership in investigations. Setting ourselves up to succeed, setting our teams up to succeed and then supporting them through what can be a difficult and emotional period will boost the likelihood of success.

When you are leading or facilitating a simple Outcome Analysis or a more detailed incident investigation, be aware of your mindset, including how you are thinking about the incident and the work being done in the investigation. There is a great opportunity to practise great leadership both before and after a workplace incident, and that will in large part be due to your mindset.

There seem to be endless shelves full of books on leadership out there, and I have read many of them. Three or four stand out for me as being especially relevant to workplace incident investigations. To me they are: *Start with Why: How Great Leaders Inspire Everyone to Take Action* by Simon Sinek, *Why Should Anyone Be Led by You? What It Takes to Be an Authentic Leader* by Rob Goffee and Gareth Jones and *Turn the Ship Around: A True Story of Turning Followers into Leaders* by L. David Marquet. *Blue Ocean Strategy: How to Create Uncontested Market Space and Make the Competition Irrelevant* by W. Chan Kim and Renee A. Mauborgne should also be thrown into the mix.

Sinek's *Start with Why* tells us that, as a leader and someone about to commence a workplace incident investigation, you need to have clarity around exactly why you are doing the investigation. You need to understand why you think it is important and why you want it to succeed. Sinek says that if you get that part of the 'why', you will become more passionate about following the process, and actively strive to understand what happened and why.

In the case of a workplace incident investigation, once that is clear, you can slip into some of the ideas explored in *Why Should Anyone Be Led by You?* The authors of this text, Goffee and Jones, talk about a number of phrases that have really struck a chord with me. These include: "Be yourself – more", "to be a leader, you must be yourself", "the context's the thing" and "great leaders are able to read the context and respond accordingly". By being yourself – driven by a deep understanding about your 'why' and leading the incident investigation team in such a way that they truly comprehend the incident – you can start to empower the incident investigation team to do their work while you are there to support their decisions, as explored in *Turn the Ship Around*. Apart from the general view regarding empowerment of the team, there are a couple of elements that Marquet talks about in *Turn the Ship Around* that pertain very much to leading and facilitating workplace incident investigations. One especially that comes to mind is the idea to "resist the urge to provide solutions"; letting and encouraging the investigation team to figure it out rather than the leader or facilitator imparting their wisdom. This can be incredibly powerful. A highly experienced leader or facilitator can easily fall into the trap of providing solutions, ideas and answers to questions. This runs the risk of losing the power of the diversity and expertise within the team. The other is encouraging the team to 'think out loud'; where conversations within the investigation team that explore their ideas and thoughts beyond the obvious are allowed to progress. Making the time and place to explore left-field discussions are not a waste of time in a detailed incident investigation.

The area where I see *Blue Ocean Strategy*'s ideas playing a role is in the methodology used for incident investigations. Kim and Mauborgne call for us to Eliminate, Reduce, Raise and Create. I have borrowed these action titles and reworked them into the incident investigation and safety space:

- **Eliminate** the prehistoric view that workers are a problem to be fixed and start seeing workers as a resource to be harnessed.
- **Reduce** the amount of hindsight bias in the conversations and the use of 'human error' as a cause for incidents.

- **Raise** the level of awareness and conversations in your organization with respect to the New View of safety.
- **Create** a new language, or way of talking about workplace incidents and safety in line with what you learn in this book.

For your consideration:

Do you challenge your peers when they express an "I already know what happened and why" attitude when they first hear about a workplace incident?

What is your first reaction when you are told about an incident in your organization? (Explore your own mindset.)

The basis of much of what is covered in this book is driven from Dekker's definition of safety as described in *Just Culture: Balancing Safety and Accountability*. In his words, safety is "the presence of positive capabilities, capacities and competencies that make things go right and not as the absence of things that go wrong". Erik Hollnagel's and Todd Conklin's descriptions of safety are very similar to this.

This definition of safety has had a profound impact on my views and thoughts on what safety is and how we should be talking about it. Contemplation of this definition drives us to explore what normally goes right to create safety, rather than just focussing on what goes wrong in an incident. It leads us to focus on the gaps between the way the work was actually done on the day of the incident and the way the work was intended to be done by the procedure, work instruction, Task Hazard Analysis (THA) or other written process requirement. It prompts us to consider the question "What is responsible for this incident?" as opposed to "Who is responsible for this incident?" It also helps us to question whether the individuals involved had the capabilities, capacities and competencies to create safety in the first place.

As a starting point for any incident investigation, we need to put ourselves into the shoes of those involved at the time of the incident and not to dwell in the land of hindsight bias that we all unconsciously love so much. We need to understand what made sense to the person at the time; what they saw, heard, felt and thought. As Jens Rasmussen is purported to have said: "If you don't understand why it made sense for people to do what they did, it is not because they were behaving really strangely, bizarrely, or erroneously, it is because your perspective is wrong." Todd

Conklin also described it well when he said that leaders have a choice when it comes to their perspectives; after a workplace incident we can either blame someone for doing something wrong, or we can learn something from what happened. We cannot do both.

As I have mentioned before, I suggest that it is not only after something goes wrong that we can learn through applying the thoughts and ideas discussed in this book. We can also apply them when things go right: I was approached a few months ago by an excited manager who said that her team had just gone 200 days without a recordable injury. She sounded very proud and seemed to be looking for some affirmation of what a great job they had done. My response deflated her a bit when I said that that was interesting but that I was more interested in how they had done it. What had they done differently over the last 200 days when compared to the time prior to the 200 days? What had changed? We talked further and in the end she was off to ask some questions and do a bit of an investigation to see if they could work out what had happened and why. It was a great conversation that included talking about learning from when things go right being just as important as learning from when things do not go right. This is very much about your mindset during the process.

For your consideration:

What does 'safety' mean to you?

How does your definition of safety impact what you look for both before and after an incident?

2 Before you investigate

Team formation, structure and roles

One of the difficulties in carrying out an effective workplace incident investigation is deciding who should be involved in the investigation team. Like many things, it is a continuum between an Outcome Analysis, which requires a small team comprising those directly and closely involved in the incident to a high-powered, manager-led and somewhat independent formal investigation team for the more detailed incident investigations. I will cover the team requirements for both levels of investigation. It is up to you to decide which will work better for the incident you are investigating at the time. As we will see, the vast majority of the thinking and science is common between the two processes.

So, who should be the members in an Outcome Analysis team? To start with, appointing the front-line supervisor or superintendent whose team was directly involved in the incident as the investigation leader is a must for the Outcome Analysis process. It has the added bonus of boosting their leadership and investigation skills and, if done well, credibility with their team. They will need support from those more senior in the organization, so it is important that senior leaders take a genuine interest in what the investigation team uncovers during the investigation. The investigation leader will need to have completed some simple Outcome Analysis training beforehand.

We also need to involve those who were at the heart of the incident – those who know what actually happened and can explain what they saw, heard and thought immediately before and during the incident. This is a bit different from the approach I use for more detailed incident investigations, where the individual involved is interviewed but does not form a part of the incident investigation team. In the case of Outcome Analyses, I find that having the people directly involved participate as core members of the investigation team really helps to uncover exactly what happened and to establish how the work is normally done as compared to whatever is in the procedure or work instruction.

Participation in the investigation team by others who carry out the same tasks as those involved in the incident (but were not directly associated with the incident) will also help enhance the team's understanding of how things normally go right, but did not go right this particular time. This is usually best achieved by using someone from another shift, ward or area of the business, as they will be familiar with the work that was being done at the time of the incident but not directly involved in it. Experience with actual investigations has shown that if you do not have this person participating in the investigation team, it is often a deal breaker and the investigation team does not get to really understand how the work is normally done outside of the area where the incident occurred. I therefore recommend that this role is a compulsory one on the team. It is also helpful to have someone who has had experience carrying out Outcome Analyses, to guide the supervisors during the incident investigations and act as an investigation facilitator.

It is often unnecessary to involve managers or safety professionals in simple Outcome Analysis investigations. In fact, I think it shows good leadership when senior leaders trust the lower-level leaders to carry out these investigations and leave them to it.

Another tip: it is best to avoid complex and interfering processes when it comes to approving the final reports of simple investigations. Keep it simple; those involved in the Outcome Analysis investigation should be as close as possible to the incident itself and they should be allowed to do their investigation work unimpeded. They know how the real world works, rather than how safety professionals and managers 'think' the world works.

Even though I have suggested their inclusion above, there has been much debate and discussion over recent years regarding whether or not the person directly involved in the incident should be a member of the workplace incident investigation team. Certainly, if the person has been significantly injured, has witnessed some nasty incident or is otherwise sensitive to the events, you will need to be very careful about their level of involvement in the incident investigation process. But in the majority of incidents that require only a simple Outcome Analysis, I strongly suggest their involvement. This not only helps them understand what happened and why, but also encourages an open, transparent and just process of incident investigation. Too many times over the last twenty years or so I have heard people complain about the investigation process being a 'black box' with statements going in one end and a written warning coming out the other end. This behaviour and perception must stop.

The fact that the story of the incident is built by the team closest to the incident is another benefit of involving the people at the centre of the incident. They do not 'get investigated' by outsiders who do not really understand how things are 'actually done around here'. They are able to work out what happened – what went right, what did not quite work out as planned and what they can do about it going forward. Ownership, participation, involvement and transparency all go a long way to a good quality investigation and, of course, a happy and productive workplace.

If a decision is made to carry out a more detailed incident investigation rather than a simple Outcome Analysis, then a broader variety of people are needed. Here is a team set-up that I have used many times and think works very well for those more detailed incident investigations.

The main person accountable for the investigation, both in terms of making sure the investigation is completed and also for its quality, is the owner of the risk. By this I mean the person who is accountable for the area in which the incident occurred. This is usually the manager of the area. I do not believe this person should be directly involved in the running of the investigation itself. They should, however, be extremely interested in it.

This 'risk owner' talks with his or her peers and identifies someone to be the investigation leader. The investigation leader for more detailed incident investigations should always be at manager level or above. I have found that if we do not front-end load the investigation team with this kind of horsepower and seniority, we will not be able to identify the truly organizational factors we strive for. I have also seen that an incident investigation leader who has some level of independence adds immense value to the output of the investigation. An independent incident investigation leader is disinterested in the detail of the incident, has no axe to grind, has nothing to hide and can provide an additional set of eyes and question sets than those closer to the incident.

Once the independent investigation leader has been nominated, we need an investigation process facilitator. This person needs to be fully trained in the incident investigation methodology, with a proven track record of being able to get the best out of a team, to *herd cats* – as the saying goes. Keeping team members focussed on their individual tasks and all roughly going in the same direction is a skill that is both rewarding and very tiring. Ensuring all members are participating, while minimizing hindsight bias, following the method process and generally keeping the team functioning are all roles for the investigation facilitator.

Both the investigation leader and the investigation facilitator need to be independent of the area or function where the incident occurred.

Team selection can make or break an investigation. You need to strike a balance between having a healthy variety of team members so that the investigation considers many views, and having too many team members, which runs the risk of becoming an uncontrollable rabble.

I once did a fatality investigation with twelve team members and found that such a number was totally unnecessary for the job at hand and a real hassle to manage and control. Even with all my experience as an incident investigation facilitator, it was extremely difficult to ensure the investigation went smoothly. Do not set yourself up to fail. Try to aim for a maximum of six people in total.

So, who should those six be? We already have an incident investigation leader and a facilitator. We need someone who understands the technical aspects of the incident. If we have had an incident that involved electricity or its supply, I would want an electrical engineer or power supply expert in the team. If the incident is a medication error-related incident, then I would want a pharmacist on the team. This team member will be able to help the rest of the team understand how the system is supposed to work, what the procedures say and the like. We also need someone who really understands how we normally do the work. So, in the electrical incident, I would have an electrician from another shift on the investigation team – one who wants to be involved and is not afraid to say how things really are. In the case of a medication error incident, I would suggest having a nurse who does similar work to that in the incident and who is from another ward or area in this role. This role is critical in helping the investigation team understand the 'Work-As-Normal' aspects.

Having a safety representative or a union rep on the team is also a good idea as these people are usually passionate about safety and can greatly help with the 'Work-As-Normal' aspects as well as freely challenging the team.

Sometimes (though not necessarily always) a safety person would also add value, especially if the incident has some level of complexity in relation to technical safety aspects. If the incident involves a contractor partner, consider replacing the safety representative or safety person with a person from the contracting company. This can be especially useful in helping understand how the contractor sets up their work processes and training.

In terms of roles, the risk owner's role is to:

- Appoint the investigation leader.
- Together with the investigation leader, appoint the facilitator.
- Approve the investigation team.
- Visit the investigation team to get updates on progress at various times throughout the investigation process, such as after timeline creation, after the team has identified differences between Work-As-Done, Work-As-Normal and Work-As-Intended, and when the organizational factors have been identified.

- Show an interest in the team and its investigation.
- Not change any aspect of the draft or final investigation report without talking with and understanding the investigation team's perspective.
- Review the quality of the investigation report.

The investigation leader's role is to:

- Set the team up for success.
- Ensure members are available when required.
- Schedule and coordinate investigation activities and resources.
- Assign duties to the team.
- Support the investigation facilitator in the process.
- Solve disagreements.
- Liaise with the risk owner on progress and outcomes.
- Supervise preparation of the investigation report (and involve the facilitator in the review of the draft report).
- Brief management on the team's findings.

The investigation facilitator's role is to:

- Facilitate the investigation process.
- Be trained and competent in applying the investigation methodology.
- Have prior experience as a facilitator (in the absence of experience, the facilitator must be coached and supported by a competent and experienced facilitator in the team, usually in the background).
- Assist the investigation leader in the review of the draft investigation report.
- Undertake routine facilitation of investigations.
- Undertake routine reviews of investigation report quality.

The investigation team member's role is to:

- Participate in all meetings and activities as directed by the investigation leader.
- Collect data, facts and information as directed.
- Establish the sequence of events leading up to the incident.
- Analyse and integrate available information.
- Analyse findings and establish conclusions.
- Participate in, and be interested in understanding what happened and why, rather than with a mindset of seeking to establish who is accountable for the incident.

The team members should not:

- Be placed in a situation of potential conflict of interest with the investigation process or findings, or
- Be there solely because they were available.

For your consideration:

Who currently leads your workplace incident investigations? (What level of management are they?)

In your investigations, do you involve those who know how the work really gets done?

The art of facilitation and using a coaching style

A critical and often overlooked skill for a facilitator of an investigation is the ability to facilitate. This may sound obvious, but it is often forgotten about or simply ignored. Facilitation is an art that eases a process, that lubricates the wheels of logic, and that helps the investigation team be the best it can be. I say it is an art as, although it can be learned, it requires adaptive thinking, generous listening and a good dose of humility to conquer well.

I have watched and listened to many people as they have participated in investigation facilitators' workshops. Some pick up the concepts of the investigation process easily and can answer any technical questions I fire at them, but have very low levels of skills when it comes to facilitation. They may understand the model well, know the theory, but do not have the control needed to keep an investigation team on track and the strength to keep it all together. When you are considering who to train as incident investigation facilitators, my advice is not to necessarily go for a technical safety person, or someone who understands your business well. Instead, go for people who are capable of facilitating groups already. All that needs to be done then is to get them up to speed with the incident investigation process and the role of the facilitator in that space.

Especially as it relates to maximizing the quality of an incident investigation, here are some skills that your facilitators should possess:

- A sound knowledge and understanding of the investigation methods and models they are using. They need to be able to explain them effectively to the incident investigation and management teams in your business.
- Listening: the ability to listen generously and to listen to understand.
- The ability to maintain the conversation amongst the investigation team.

- Control the disclosure of their viewpoint unless asked.
- Remember that the incident investigation is all about the team, not about them as the facilitator.
- Control the level and direction of the conversations during the incident investigation.
- Ask questions in different ways.
- Involve everybody in the conversation and not allow strong characters in the investigation team to dominate.

One point is worth going into a bit more detail here, and that is the last one: "Involve everybody in the conversation and not allow strong characters in the investigation team to dominate". As you are facilitating, it is important to involve everybody in the team. A mixture of levels, skills sets, backgrounds and levels of willingness are all at your disposal. Use them. The diversity in an investigation team is what can make the difference between an OK investigation and a brilliant one.

Some investigation team members may also simply dislike talking in front of others, or feel their contribution is not worthwhile. An important part of the facilitator's job is to keep everybody involved – to invite people to speak up if they are quiet, to challenge those who talk a lot, to find a way to let others add their thoughts to the conversation, and to generally make everyone in the incident investigation team feel safe and secure enough to talk about and contribute whatever they want. Do not allow others to put people down or talk over others. Keep absolute control of the conversations. If there is a side conversation stop it immediately, even if it is a senior manager taking the lead in that distraction. The role of the facilitator is often one of balance and art rather than process and application. It is by far the most difficult job in the investigation team. In many ways, the art of the facilitator is closely related to the art of coaching.

There is a wonderful opportunity to bring a non-directive coaching style into investigations for this reason. In order to do this, we need to explore what coaching is and what a coaching model could look like within the context of a workplace incident investigation. In his brilliant book *Effective Coaching: Lessons from the Coach's Coach*, Myles Downey describes coaching as "the art of facilitating the performance, learning and development of another". I feel that coaching fits perfectly within the investigation space.

In the case of an incident investigation, I feel it is legitimate to translate Downey's definition of coaching into: "the art of facilitating the performance of the incident investigation team – to be the best it can be".

A noble goal of a facilitator is to help the incident investigation team adopt a learning and listening attitude during the interview and data-gathering steps of the investigation. And if coaching is all about asking questions to seek understanding (which it is!) you can use a coaching style to support and facilitate the performance of the investigation team, especially when team members are carrying out interviews. You will certainly have a better quality investigation if you succeed in achieving this goal. One of the ways to end up with a hindsight bias-filled, pre-ordained outcome in your investigation report is to have a facilitator who has an agenda; a facilitator who already knows what has caused the incident, knows the answers to questions before they have been asked and has strong opinions about the incident. At the other end of the scale, having an investigation facilitator who applies a coaching style minimizes this for the betterment of understanding the incident – by giving due attention to the engagement, inclusion, full participation and development of the investigation team. It is also a good reason to ensure that any facilitator you use for an investigation is not from the area where the incident has occurred.

Coaching styles can range from the more 'directive' approaches of telling, instructing or giving advice through guidance and feedback, to making suggestions in a more 'non-directive' style – i.e. asking questions to focus, raise awareness and listen to understand.

So, what could coaching look like during an incident investigation? Whether you are a front-line supervisor or a more senior manager, those investigating workplace incidents need to be very interested in understanding how the work is normally done and what went differently on the day of the incident. Using a mainly non-directive coaching style to ask questions can make a huge difference in helping us gain a solid understanding of these issues. It is also a style that is non-threatening and has the sole aim of helping the team, not providing the answers.

A common coaching style uses the GROW model (see Figure 2.1) and is one that lends itself to use during incident investigations. This is the model described well in *Effective Coaching: Lessons from the Coach's Coach* by Myles Downey. GROW is an acronym. It stands for Goal, Reality, Options and Wrap-up, or Will-do. During the early part of a pure coaching conversation the purpose or goal (G) is set. This is normally the purpose of the coaching interaction. In the case of an incident this is pretty much established as the reason for the investigation itself. If you were feeling pedantic, you could set the goal as "To explore and understand the workplace incident and to establish what we can learn from it". The Reality of the present state is then explored, Options are teased out and then commitments are made (Wrap-up/Will-do). And how is all of this achieved? Through the use of questions asked by the coach, and then the coach listening to the answers given by the player. (In the case of a workplace incident investigation, this is the investigation team.)

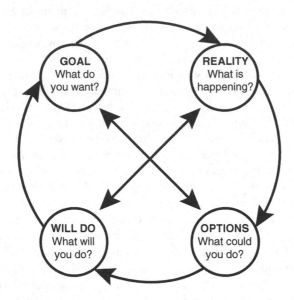

Figure 2.1 The GROW model

The two elements of the GROW model that are most useful to us during an incident investigation are the Reality element and the Options element. Let's focus on using Reality in an investigation to start with.

Imagine that you are out in the plant, or on the ward, having a conversation with a work team about how they normally do their work. This could be as part of an incident investigation or it could be as part of your normal day-to-day leadership activities. Now, the 'Reality' bit of coaching is all about getting an accurate picture of the way things are – so we need to remember not to pass judgement about what we are told, rather to simply gather the information we need. This means no analysing, criticizing, jumping to conclusions, and no trying to fix or solve something. Our job at this stage is to understand how the teams normally carry out this work on a day-to-day basis. It is about getting to an understanding of what the 'reality' is for those doing the work. Analysing how work is done against a procedure or process is a separate activity that we will explore at a later stage.

Another opportunity to use a coaching style is when the investigation team is trying to come to terms with the various factors that contributed to the incident. The facilitator can bring additional focus to the investigation team by using both the Reality and the Options parts of the GROW model. This is where the facilitator asks questions exploring how things happened and how they normally happen as the team reviews the information collected during the data-gathering component of the investigation, removing any supposition, assumptions and guesswork. As they explore corrective actions at a later stage of the investigation, the facilitator moves to Options and often asks: "What else could we do?" "What else do we need to see?"

Even if the facilitator is far more experienced than those on the team, applying a coaching style to all their work will help the team reach a better landing on their story about what happened and why than when the facilitator suggests answers to their own rhetorical questions.

Here are some questions that may help a facilitator use a coaching style in an incident investigation. They are intended to inform a conversation rather than to be asked directly as they are written.

Reality
What happened then?
Who has got the information about how this task is normally done?
What exactly does the procedure say about this?
How many times did they do that in the last week/month?
When was the last time that happened?
Who else was involved in the situation, and how?
Which factors are most important here?
What makes you say that?
Tell me more.
You mentioned that _____. Can you say more about that?
Give me some background: what led to your having that view?
What's behind that?
Who else has some information in relation to this?
What have you got?
What else fed into this?
What does this look like from the other person's point of view?
Give me a specific example of that.
What exactly did they say?
OK – so run through that from square one. Exactly what happened?
Say more about that.
Keep going.
Tell me more.
What else?
And?
Give me a concrete example of that.

Options
What did you mean when you said _____?
Let's shoot for at least five potential reasons. What else do we have?

What could we do to overcome this? What are our options?

What other resources could we draw on to tackle this?

What other options can you think of?

You mentioned earlier that _____. Does that suggest any other ways we could approach this?

The options we have mentioned so far are [read back through the list of options the team has generated]. What stands out in that list?

What would it look like to conquer this once and for all?

Give me five options for how we could tackle this challenge.

Give me another option.

What else could we do?

What do we need that we don't have right now?

Who do you know that could help us with this?

Wrap up/Will do

Which wording do we want to settle on?

Are we all happy with this?

Turn that into an action step: what will we ask who to do by when?

On a scale of one to ten, how likely is it that this step will get us where we need to be?

Are there any obstacles we need to address to make sure this action gets done?

Is that a realistic story? Does it all hold together and make sense?

For your consideration:

Does your organization support coaching and the use of the GROW model?

Do you use a coaching style during problem-solving, mentoring and during workplace incident investigations?

How many of the questions above and in the appendices have you asked before or during an incident investigation or when you were interviewing someone after a workplace incident?

Your conversations and questions (before and after an event)

"The conversations we have before an incident should be the same as the conversations we have after an incident." I have said this often and will continue to do so as I believe it is a cornerstone of not only investigations but also 'safety' leadership generally. Both in a workplace incident investigation after an incident and also in the field on a day-to-day basis as a great 'safety' leader, we should be interested in the same things and hence have the same conversations. In an incident investigation, we are trying to understand the gaps between the way work was done on the day of the incident (Work-As-Done), how others normally do the work (Work-As-Normal) and how our processes and procedures intended it to be done (Work-As-Intended); and then we work to understand what lies behind these gaps and close them. That is fine and normal after an incident, but what about before an incident? When we are out and about on the ward, in the production plant or underground in the mine we are, or at least should be, trying to understand the gaps between the way work was done on the day we were out there being a visible leader (Work-As-Done), how others normally do the work (Work-As-Normal) and how our processes and procedures intended it to be done (Work-As-Intended); and then we work to close the gaps we have identified during the conversations. "The conversations we have before an incident should be the same as the conversations we have after an incident." So, I encourage you to remember this quote and think about it both before, and after, a workplace incident.

For your consideration:

Spend some time out in your business over the next few weeks on a journey of discovery. Look for and understand how work is actually done, and see if it is exactly the same as how you might think it is being done (as per the procedures and systems).

Think about whether you are OK with the fact that the real world does not always match the world contained within procedures and work instructions. Explore your own behaviour here, before looking at those around you. Do you always follow all the procedures in your business?

3   The investigation process

Scene preservation

In many ways, this part of a workplace incident investigation is not part of the investigation at all. In the vast majority of circumstances, the need to preserve the scene occurs when the incident investigation team has not yet been formed. It is usually left up to the local area leadership to preserve the scene and make everything safe.

Subsequent to the initiation of the site emergency or field response plan, and the implementation of any immediate corrective actions necessary to prevent escalation of the incident (or to prevent further incidents from occurring), a critical step in the pre-work needed before an incident investigation process is formally commenced is scene preservation and early data-gathering. This step, which is often very poorly done, can have an enormous impact on the quality of the investigation. An absence of data and information can very effectively stall the investigation. The amount of time, effort and resources spent on scene preservation will vary considerably depending on the level and complexity of the incident itself. The list below may only be completed in its entirety for a fatal incident or a potentially fatal incident. I have put an asterisk next to the elements that are an absolute minimum for Outcome Analyses and other similar simple incident investigations.

Before looking at the list, I'd like to share with you two of the fatality investigations that I have facilitated to show the difference between a well-done and a poorly done scene preservation, and how they impacted the investigations. The first fatality was related to two mining haul trucks that collided, killing one of the operators. The investigation team arrived on the scene about two days after the tragic incident and not only had the operation secured the immediate scene, but also the haul road ramp above the incident for some hundreds of metres. Because the scene was so well preserved, the investigation team was able to discern the areas where the haul truck operator had attempted to control the vehicle (through repeated application of the retarder brake as it drove down the hill). This greatly helped us form a view of what led to the incident.

The other incident occurred when a front-end loader dropped a bucket full of material onto the head of an operator who was busy cleaning out a material transfer chute in a mine in South Africa. I visited the site on the day of the incident and noticed a cleaning sparge and air hose draped over the lip of the chute. The sparge was quite short and it was surmised that this could have been one of the reasons why the operator was inside the chute rather than cleaning the chute from a platform adjacent to the open top of the chute. The scene was locked down and the team was to convene at the site early the next morning once the rest of the investigation team arrived at the site. Strict instructions were given to ensure that nobody touched anything overnight. When the complete team assembled and visited the scene the following morning, we noticed the sparge was now its full length of approximately 2 metres. A member of the incident investigation team asked why the operator did not stand on the platform to clean the chute. I pointed out that someone had changed the sparge overnight and the one that was there the previous night was far shorter. This was confirmed by looking at photographs taken at the time of the incident. If I had not visited the scene the day before, the investigation team would not have been aware of this and confusion, supposition and guesswork would have prevailed during the investigation process.

There are two ways to ensure early scene preservation. One is ensuring that your front-line supervisors are fully aware of the importance of scene preservation and the role the supervisor can play. The second is making a quick decision on the level of the investigation that you plan to carry out, and then sending people to the scene early to capture vital data and information.

Here are some simple but absolutely essential activities to consider. As I mentioned above, the items with an asterisk are essential for all levels of incident investigation, with the others optional other than for a detailed serious or even fatality-level event, where they are needed:

- * Get to the scene as soon as possible after the incident. Try to be there before physical evidence is disturbed.
- Do not pre-judge the situation.
- * Make an assessment of the level of incident investigation that is required.
- Do not move or remove anything,
  - ask if anybody else has moved or removed anything.
- * Take photographs – distance shots, close-ups, all at different angles, taking notes of each photo, as well as a panoramic shot of the total area.
- Take videos.

- Draw sketches, including distances.
- Take measurements.
- * Identify people who may have information that needs to be captured early and carry out preliminary interviews (do not simply take statements).
- Note the lighting.
- Note the weather.
- Note the working conditions.
- Note the housekeeping.
- Record what tools and equipment are at the scene.
- If you attempt any re-creations, think about what you are trying to achieve before getting stuck into the task. Do a formal risk assessment and have all the questions you are seeking answers to in place before the re-enactment takes place. I have seen too many injuries during incident re-enactments due to poor planning and poor thinking.

For your consideration:

Who is accountable for incident preservation in your organization?

Do your current training systems for front-line supervisors cover what to do in the event of a workplace incident?

Does your incident investigation procedure or guideline outline what to do to preserve the scene of an incident?

Interviewing (versus taking statements)

Over the more than twenty years that I have been working in the field of occupational health and safety, my job has taken me to many different parts of the world – I've lived and worked in Australia, South Africa, Mozambique, Chile, Suriname, and I have also facilitated fatality investigations in the United States and the Democratic Republic of Congo.

No matter which country I am in when running an investigation, I've found there is a tendency for managers to believe that there is a legal requirement for investigation teams to take 'statements' from those involved in incidents and to also take statements from those who may have seen what transpired during an incident. You may have noticed that I did not use the phrase 'witnessed the incident' in the last sentence. It may sound pedantic but the use of words like 'witness', 'evidence' and 'procedural breach' all hint of a crime, an incident for which we need to identify the guilty party. The statements that are then taken too often become the backbone of an investigation and are sometimes used to 'hold people accountable' for their decisions, words and actions, when in reality all we are looking for is their story.

I have generally found that a legal requirement to take statements does not exist. I suggest you chat with your legal team about this. And if you have the requirement to take statements in your safety or human resources systems, remove them. Moreover, I urge you to stop asking people to provide them. I have a strong opinion about statements, and that is that they are toxic.

Let me explain why I am so strongly opposed to the taking of statements. Generally speaking, the people who may see or be involved in an incident will not be a Shakespeare, or a Tolkien, they will not be poet laureates, nor are they likely to be regular bloggers or vloggers. They will tend not to create a 5,000-word tome explaining their feelings about the incident, including their observations, sensory inputs, visual clues, inner emotions and other details that led up to that moment. Nor are they likely to list the specific details of all of their procedural 'breaches' for you. Instead, they are likely to write down as little as possible – and that is mainly just to get you off their back.

If you are lucky, you may get two paragraphs stating the obvious. The writers of the statement will also tend to lean towards something that does not self-incriminate. Likewise, they will hardly ever dob in their mates (translated from Australian: will not get their workmates into trouble), nor will they always give you all that you are looking for. This last point is extremely important. People will tend to write down what they think you want to hear. If your organization is still one of the archaic ones that prefers to find out *who* is responsible for an incident rather than *what* is responsible, then you will not get much information about what people did or did not do, simply out of fear. Having a conversation is far more powerful.

Other problems concerning statements and interviews emerge that relate to the psychology of writing, learning and memory. Many of us aid our learning by writing things down. I certainly do. In fact, when I read a technical book or listen to a technical podcast, I tend to summarize it in words. I often find that I have a thirty- or forty-page summary of a book that I have read. It helps me to learn. A lecture theatre at university is the perfect place to see this in action; hundreds of students all with their heads down, madly scribbling away. They are helping cement their knowledge. It's important to remember that the act of writing helps to create memory, and once a memory has been built in this fashion, it is often very difficult for it to change. Usually what people involved in the incident write down will become the facts as they recall them. They are also not likely to change their story away from what they wrote in the first instance, for fear of being accused of fabricating the truth. I have seen this happen a lot, where a person does not want to change the story as they wrote it down in their statement. Even if the story in their statement does not make any logical or physical sense.

For all of these reasons, having a guided conversation with those involved in the incident leaves us so much better off. If you like, you can perceive this conversation as an interview, with the interviewer capturing whatever data is shared for future use in the investigation.

Do not ask them to sign the document. Do not get them to approve the document. The information you have written down is simply for your use. A set of notes if you like. Those notes are your own synopsis of what you both talked about during the interview. They are not a formal record. They should not be something that will go on the individual's human resources department record. At the end of the day, it is a bit like a meeting. We all take notes at a meeting but we would not generally read the notes back to the meeting, or make other people sign off on the notes, as if checking to make sure we have captured their comments perfectly. We all take notes to capture information and ideas for our own needs, what we perceived has gone on during a meeting. My recommendation is to take a similar approach here. You are having a conversation with someone for the purposes of getting a better understanding of their story. It is as simple as that. Okay. If you still haven't got the message and if you currently take statements, and intend to continue to do so, STOP IT.

Now, let's talk about how to have a good and powerful conversation while gathering data for the investigation (I think conversation is a much better word than interview).

Before getting into the technical details of what to say and how to say it, remember what we are there for: to better understand a person's story about a series of events. We are not there as a means to get information that is owed to us. We need to set up our mind to listen generously. And we need to set up the conversation so that it happens as soon after the incident as possible. Memories fade and are altered far more quickly and permanently than we realize.

For your consideration:

Do you take statements, have formal interviews or have conversations to gather data and information for your workplace incident investigations?

During your next incident investigations try having some conversations, instead of taking statements.

Before we look at the 'how to' in any depth, let's examine generous listening a bit more.

Generous listening

The ability of people to listen seems not to have changed much over the last twenty or so years. Or at least I have not noticed much of an improvement. Everyone wants to have their say, is intent on interrupting and not listening to what is actually being said.

Generous listening is an art. It is an art that needs constant attention and practice. It is the art of using your whole body and self in the act of listening. It is about listening to understand rather than listening to respond. It is about paying attention to what is going on behind or within the words. It is not about the person doing the listening. It is about the person being listened to. In this vein, the questions being asked are very important. However, the way in which these questions are being asked is more important.

Think of the process of gathering information from those involved in a workplace incident as a conversation, rather than a list of questions that must be answered, or as a formal interview. That said, you will of course need to ask some questions; it is how you ask them that makes the difference. I have included a list of questions in Appendix A that I have found helpful in the past. This list may also help you think about some topics that may be of interest during the information-gathering process. I use this list each and every time I facilitate an incident investigation – not all of it of course, but I do scan it and select some key question topics pertinent to the incident being investigated. It helps get my mind in the right space for the conversations I'm about to have in the data- and information-gathering stage of the investigation.

I have heard it said, as I am sure you have, that we have two ears and one mouth and that we should use them in that ratio. I prefer a ratio of five to one. Listen five times more than you speak when you are having an incident-related conversation with someone.

It takes a fair amount of time and effort to practise generous listening. Here are a few things to focus on: Listen not only to what is being said but also to what is being left unsaid. Are the verbal and non-verbal messages in conflict, or are they congruent? Is the person saying something that just doesn't 'seem' to match the way it is being said, or the facial or body language with which it is being said? In the world of communication, you can either talk or you can listen. Do not try to do both at once; it is not possible. The next time you are having a conversation with a friend and they are telling you something, start talking to them about something else and see if you can still listen to them *and* keep track of what your friend is talking about. It is not possible – unless you have the skills of a simultaneous translator.

If you are having a conversation with someone in order to find out more about an incident, and whilst they are talking you interrupt, you have done a couple of major things wrong. One is that you have stopped them talking and hence you have stopped them thinking. You have also interrupted your flow of listening, and as I have said before, it is not possible to listen and talk at the same time, so just be quiet and listen.

In summary, then, there are a number of things that we should try to focus on when listening and talking during an interview. They are:

- Listen, and stop talking.
- Be prepared for the conversation. Go through Appendix A and think about the topics you would like to hear more about during the conversation. Put other elements that are at risk of distracting both you and the other person out of your mind.
- Prepare the person you are having the conversation with by helping them be at ease. Remind them that this is just an information-gathering activity, similar to a meeting, and not some formal human resources or legal process.
- Take notes just as you would in any meeting.
- Be truly empathetic to the feelings of the person you are talking with. They may be nervous and uncertain. Try to stand in their shoes and see the issues and actions from their perspective.
- Use your body language to support the person. Cues are useful here, so nod or use short words of encouragement. Stay focussed on the person. Maintain appropriate eye contact.
- Be patient. Do not argue. Silence is a great tool to use. Let the person take as much time as they need to corral their thoughts and words.
- Remove distractions from the environment. Turn your cell phone off. Don't shuffle papers, don't check email and don't keep looking at whoever is walking past or your watch.
- Never be judgemental. Simply listen to understand.
- Listen beyond the words. Listen to the tone, and the alignment between the words and body language. Listen for what is not being said as well as what is being said.

We all have a little voice inside our heads. Some of the things that little voice says to us as we listen can include:

- So what?
- I'm bored.

- I know EXACTLY what you did... and it is not what you are telling me right now.
- What should I ask next?
- I have heard all this before.
- Come on!
- Hurry up and answer the question I asked you.
- You are evading my questions.
- I'm hungry.
- He looks really nervous. He must be lying.

Watch out for these and try not to listen to them. This is sometimes difficult, but generous listening is not always easy, and in fact is actually hard work and often tiring. Yet, the benefits are vast.

> **For your consideration:**
>
> Next time you are in a meeting or in a conversation with a number of people, explore how you are listening.
>
> Try setting up a 'listening coach' role in your next routine meeting.
>
> Watch yourself in your next few conversations. Are you listening to respond or are you listening to understand?

The interview conversation

Once we are ready to start the conversation, thinking about and then adopting these three simple approaches will yield a wealth of information:

1. Free recall – narrative: this entails allowing the person you are having the conversation with (i.e. interviewing) to give you an idea of what they can recall. Ask them to tell their story. That is the best way to start the interview. In fact, this should be in relation to the general "how work is normally done here" conversation rather than starting at the part of the conversation that relates to the day of the incident. As they open up, just close your mouth and listen. Listen generously. Listen with your eyes, with your body and with your mind.

2. Open questions: these are questions that cannot be answered with a simple, "yes" or "no" or any other single words, but are designed so that the person continues to share information with you. Examples

are things like: "Tell me what happened after that", "How do you normally react when that happens?"

3. Closed questions (including multiple choice): these are questions that are designed to limit the responses available to the interviewee. These questions are best for following up on a response to an open question and can usually be answered with a single word or short answer. They are used when limited or more specific information is required. An example would be "What time did you start work after lunch?"

Do not use any form of leading questions or ask questions with the mindset that you already know the answer. For example, a question not to ask would be "You normally use a screwdriver for this job, don't you?" It is also important to have these conversations as soon after the incident as possible because any delays in conducting interviews can affect the quality and quantity of information gathered.

Human memories are fallible and impermanent. They fade quickly and are heavily impacted by the views and conversations we have with others. We want to minimize as much as possible those involved getting together and chatting before you have a chance to talk with them. A group of people will quickly establish 'one way' that the incident occurred and it will become part of their collective memory and story. I saw an example of this many years ago when a person fell into a piece of machinery in a steel mill. The supervisor got the team together and tried to understand the incident. The person with the loudest opinion ended up convincing all the others about what they all saw. Even though the story as they all told it afterwards was not possible, they all vehemently believed that is what they saw.

Sometimes it is beneficial to have the interview conversations at the location of the incident. Visual prompts can often help people clarify what they saw or heard and it can also help them explain how they normally do the work. Be careful with this tactic, however – if there has been a fatality or serious injury, for instance, we need to be very mindful of how vivid recall can affect those who see such incidents.

As I mentioned earlier, the information you collect is for the investigation, not for some legal purpose and so it is not necessary for the individual being interviewed to read your notes or sign off on them as a fair and accurate representation. They are simply the notes you took from a conversation you had – just like you would have during any typical meeting. I have seen them called 'conversation notes' and that can help to diffuse any blame culture that may rear its ugly head during the process. Use drawings and sketches as well if it helps you make sense of the incident.

Don't forget to explain that the interview is just a conversation, or a meeting, to see what information they may have that may help sort out what work normally looks like and what happened on the day of the incident.

A few points to remember to ensure you are interviewing with purpose:

- Listen to understand.
- Listen to learn.
- Remember how you plan to use the data you are collecting (this affects the sort of data you collect and the details).
- Interview respectfully.
- Be aware of the position of people during the conversation to help facilitate a relaxed atmosphere.

By 'position of people', I mean setting up the environment in which you are having the conversation in such a way that it feels comfortable and it is clearly not an interrogation. A classic method here is the triangle. In the triangle method, there are three roles: the interviewer, the interviewee and the scribe, who is usually busy taking notes. Set up your triangle so that the interviewee is facing the interviewer with the scribe off to one side. This works as the main focus of the interviewee is always on the person asking the questions and not on both people. This helps the interviewee feel that this is not a two-on-one activity.

In the case of a detailed investigation there is a critical rule to always follow when gathering information through a conversation or an interview; it is to never carry out the interview with more than one person being interviewed at a time. Our memories are so fallible and able to be manipulated that you can end up with one story, or one version of the incident but that version may well not be true or even possible. Do any interviews quickly and in isolation of others.

All of the above applies just as validly if you are undertaking a simple Outcome Analysis or a more detailed incident investigation. In an Outcome Analysis, the conversations will be between the investigation team members as they explore how work was done and how it is normally done. In the case of a detailed investigation, the conversations are usually held before the investigation team builds a timeline and does the analysis.

There are times when a safety incident investigation is done under legal professional privilege. Different rules apply then and you should be guided by your legal advisors with respect to interviews, conversations and the gathering of information.

For your consideration:

How do you currently carry out interviews?

During the next workplace incident interview you do, or participate in, explore the balance between free recall, open and closed questions.

Data- and information-gathering

A formal data- and information-gathering step is usually reserved for the more detailed incident investigations. In a simple Outcome Analysis, this step is simply done with the team in front of a white board or around a table. The remainder of this section applies for the more detailed incident investigation process.

Conversations, as described above, can occur at any time in an investigation – usually in the very early stages but also as part of the data- and information-gathering step described here. It is worth going through how to run this step before we move on to timeline preparation.

The term we use for this step is commonly called a PEEPO. It is simply an acronym that describes the categories of data and information that we wish to collect. A PEEPO is used to help an investigation team think about what information, data and records they wish to collect – to help them understand what happened in an incident. The data buckets we use are:

People,
Environment,
Equipment,
Procedures/documentation and
Organization.

These work well as category buckets and are useful tools to jog memory. They shouldn't be seen as formal sections that must be filled.

Carrying out a PEEPO is one of the simplest tasks that needs to be carried out by the incident investigation team. You need a white board and some small sticky notes, commonly known as Post-it® notes. I implore you not to use a computer for this task as I really think it slows everything down. Computers are sequential and not simultaneous. If you use a computer, there is one poor person doing the typing and every time they misspell a word they have the rest of the team stopping to spell-check or correct them. In addition, only one idea is captured at a time and you cannot easily get a simple overview of the PEEPO in its entirety. It also runs the risk of a lack of involvement by the team.

How to run an effective and efficient PEEPO

You should have a diverse team already mobilized around you. The secret to creating a great PEEPO and a great investigation more generally is to use that diversity to your advantage. I do this during a PEEPO by distributing the blank Post-it® notes amongst the team and then asking them to jot down any information they would like to see under any of the PEEPO categories.

A great way to encourage them is to ask something like:

> Okay. Jim, you are a safety rep [or a nurse or electrician or whatever]. What is it you would like to see that would help you understand exactly what happened here, and just as importantly, how it happened, and also what was going on in the background that led to it happening? What do you want to see?

Ask them to write down the piece of information they would like to see collected onto a Post-it® note, and then get them to stick the note up on the white board under PEEP or O. Once completed (give it about 20 minutes), you will have a white board full of little Post-it® notes which you can then group into topics and which can then be distributed amongst the team (see Figure 3.1). As an example, all of the Post-it® notes that relate to maintenance can be grouped together and handed to the mechanic. Even though they could vary from maintenance records, procedures and organizational hierarchies, it just makes sense for one person to collect them together. Similarly, in a patient safety-related incident, all of the information related to the medication and its delivery might be collected together and given to a pharmacist to collect. When I'm carrying out a PEEPO like this, I then inform each member of the team that they are accountable for collecting the data and bringing it all back with them when the team reconvenes to complete the process of the investigation. The timing of that next session should be set with the investigation leader, taking into account the complexity and time constraints for the collection of the information from the PEEPO.

This first investigation team meeting ends with each team member leaving the room armed with a little collection of Post-it® notes. This

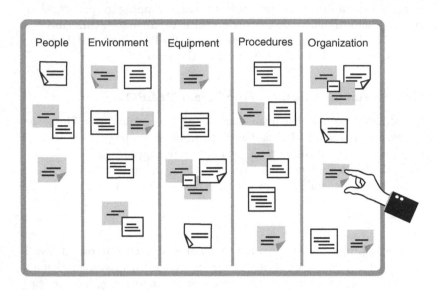

Figure 3.1 PEEPO

'collecting of the information' step usually takes in the order of a week to be completed for a detailed incident investigation.

It can be tempting to allow the safety team or the local supervisor to collect a common set of information for each and every incident and then for the investigation team to start their process using this previously collected data and information. I have seen this time and again and have developed a strong view against the practice. When supplied with data, most teams will make do with what they are given even though significant information may be missing. Once the team starts working they tend to forget that there may be more information out there and they do not always want to halt the process in order to collect it. They also do not have ownership of the collected data.

Having *all* the incident investigation team members decide for themselves what information *they* want to see and then collecting it themselves gives them a much higher level of understanding of that information and a much higher level of involvement in the investigation process. If your site has prepared a pile of information for you, then keep it to one side during the PEEPO and do not allow the team to review any of it until they have completed their PEEPO. Only then should they be allowed to check and see whether the data they want has already been supplied.

Another useful resource for the team to use once they have slowed down their Post-it® note-writing activities is Appendix A. Although Appendix A is set up as a set of questions, it can be used as a prompt list for your PEEPO. It is, however, important to allow the team to come up with most of the PEEPO on their own before exploring Appendix A, otherwise it becomes more like a checklist.

For your consideration:

What process do you currently use to decide what data and information your investigation teams need?

Who gets to decide what information an investigation team needs?

Determining Work-As-Done, Work-As-Normal and Work-As-Intended

I have intentionally broken this section into two parts. The first describes the process we use for determining Work-As-Done, Work-As-Normal and Work-As-Intended for Outcome Analyses and the second part covers the process we use for determining Work-As-Done, Work-As-Normal and Work-As-Intended for more detailed incident investigations.

There are some really important common elements, however. In both cases we should be very interested in learning and understanding how the work is actually being done and comparing it to how we might think work is being done according to procedures, work instructions and checklists.

I had the opportunity of recently observing nurses running through pre-procedure checklists at two hospitals in Perth, Western Australia from the perspective of an interested observer (patient). It was interesting to compare and contrast the two hospitals. The visits were within a month of each other with one hospital being a private hospital and the other being a public hospital and the procedure was identical (femoral angiogram and angioplasty). In the public hospital, the seemingly exhaustive checklist was meticulously completed. When I asked the nurse what she thought about the checklist and whether she felt it was important and added value, I got a resounding positive response and I observed behaviour that supported that. A month later, at the private hospital, I witnessed a very different approach. The checklists were very similar if not identical and the medical procedure was the same. That is where the similarities ended. I observed a much more lackadaisical approach to completing the checklist with some questions being answered by the nurse, questions skipped over and a general lack of interest in the process. When I asked the nurse about the level of value of the checklist, I got a "Sorry, we need to fill these out." "Half of these questions are not relevant for your procedure. We will just skip through those." With a sample size of two, I certainly did not have any evidence to suggest a difference between private and public hospitals in Australia but rather felt it represented a typical difference between two individuals and how they actually do their work. I am sure the management of the hospitals in question have a common view of how the checklists 'should' be used. This is a classic example of the difference between Work-As-Done and Work-As-Intended.

In an Outcome Analysis we do not build a detailed timeline in the traditional sense. We build a simple timeline and then focus on those 'events' that highlight the differences between how the work was done during the incident and how we thought the work was going to be done according to the procedures, work instruction or other 'safety' systems. So, before building any kind of timeline for an Outcome Analysis, or thinking about what might have gone 'wrong' in an incident, we need to find out about how the real world works. This includes how we think it works and what usually goes 'right' in the workplace on a day-to-day basis. To start this process, the supervisor or superintendent (i.e. the person we have appointed as the investigation leader) needs to become familiar with the Work-As-Intended; the way work is intended to be done in the workplace.

We can usually get a good idea of the Work-As-Intended by looking at our systems, including our work instructions, THAs, job safety analyses, procedures and standards, along with any other documented processes. These documents outline how management expects or at least wants workers to get the job done safely, effectively and efficiently.

I strongly suggest an incident investigation leader collects all the procedures and other system requirements and goes through them in detail before the investigation starts. All too commonly, supervisors are confident that they know how the work should have been done and what the procedures say, so they don't gather the procedures or go through them in enough detail for the investigation. To me, this is a big mistake. Supervisors, superintendents and other managers are just as likely to be unaware of, or omit, procedural specifics as workers are.

I like to use the example of an electrician, working at height, in a confined space with a boilermaker next to them using a gas axe to cut through a pipe. I wonder how many procedures the electrician needs to comply with in order to get the job done. I then wonder how likely it is that all of the procedures, permits, standards, trainings and other guidance material coordinate, are aligned and fit together. The likelihood that all the ducks line up between the procedures will be very close to zero.

Do not start with an analysis of the incident itself, but rather build a common story about "how we normally do this work" at the same time as building the simple timeline (or Work-As-Done). I have seen that the best results are achieved when the investigation team simply has a conversation around a white board. The informality often relaxes the team members and gets them to open up and talk about their work as it is normally done – rather than being tense and worried about what went wrong and the consequences that may be coming their way, as can happen when they are confronted with a form to fill out and sign.

Why would we want to focus on Work-As-Normal as well as Work-As-Done? We could simply look at what went wrong, try to understand why it went wrong and then fix it, couldn't we? Well, this may work in some incidents, but it will not create the mindset and forward-looking learning that we are seeking to create when carrying out an Outcome Analysis.

We need to understand that work happens the same way regardless of whether the outcome is safe work or an incident. Usually, things go right and only very rarely do they go wrong. Our role in investigations is to use 'how things normally go right' as the basis for working out 'why they did not go right this time'. This is a far more interesting and effective approach to investigations than just focussing on what went wrong. And it helps create an excellent culture of learning.

The historical view of safety was that as long as you followed the procedures religiously, or at least rigorously (i.e. "adherence to procedures is king"), you would not get hurt. However, the latest conversations in the literature strongly suggest this is not remotely how the real world works. In fact, it is uncommon for procedures to be followed precisely with all the Is dotted and Ts crossed. In the vast majority of cases our people are creating safety for themselves while they carry out their work; based on their capabilities, competencies and capacities. Moreover, they adapt to suit the conditions on the day and at the time the work is being carried out. The way the work is done in the field on a day-to-day basis rarely matches the procedure. Yet it nearly always results in 'safe work'.

By way of example, think about a set of pedestrian crossing lights in the town or city where you live or where you are reading this book. Now, there are laws in the majority of countries that I have lived and/ or worked in that require us to stop and wait on the curb when the pedestrian crossing light is red – usually depicted by a little red pictogram of a person with their arms and legs apart. We cross the road when the sign changes to a little green person that looks like they are walking. This is how the work is *intended* to be completed safely (Work-As-Intended).

If you spend five or ten minutes watching any intersection in nearly any city, you will not always see the work being done (i.e. crossing the road) according to the work as it is intended to be completed (i.e. waiting for the little red person to change to a little green person before crossing the road). Instead, you will see a variety of behaviours – ranging from completely ignoring the lights and people crossing whenever they want to, to some combination of adherence to the law and carrying out of a risk assessment before breaking the law and crossing the lights on red.

It is the same at work. Work-As-Done is the way work is actually carried out in the field, on the day of interest. It is nearly always different from Work-As-Intended, which is the way the procedure or work instruction says to do the job, and could be the same or different to how the people normally do the work (Work-As-Normal).

This is the basis of the Outcome Analysis process; the idea that the way work is actually done differs from the way managers think the work is being done every single day. We need to be extremely interested in what is driving the gaps between Work-As-Done, Work-As-Normal and Work-As-Intended, both as leaders on a day-to-day basis and also as an investigation team after an incident.

The theories behind the concepts of Work-As-Done and Work-As-Intended (or Work-As-Imagined) come from the work of Erik Hollnagel. He brilliantly describes the importance of understanding how work is normally done (no adverse outcome) as a precursor to understanding what went wrong in a passage concerning Sherlock Holmes in *Safety I and Safety II*:

> The difficulty of perceiving that which goes right can be illustrated by a conversation between Sherlock Holmes and Inspector Gregory from Scotland Yard. Among the fictional detectives, Sherlock Holmes was famous for noticing things that others either did not see, or saw but found insignificant. The conversation can be found in the short story, "Silver Blaze", which focuses on the disappearance of a famous racehorse on the eve of an important race and on the apparent murder of its trainer. During the investigation, the following conversation takes place: Gregory (a Scotland Yard detective): "Is there any other point to which you would wish to draw my attention?" Sherlock Holmes: "To the curious incident of the dog in the night-time." Gregory: "The dog did nothing in the night-time." Sherlock Holmes: "That was the curious incident." The point here is that you can only notice – and know – that something is wrong if you know

what should have happened in the everyday case. The understanding of how something is normally done (everyday work) is a necessary prerequisite for understanding whether something is (potentially) wrong. In this example Sherlock Holmes realised that a dog would normally bark when encountering a strange person. Since the dog had not barked (the "curious incident"), the person who had entered the stable (and abducted Silver Blaze) had, therefore, not been a stranger.

So, at this stage, we should know the Work-As-Intended and we have a good understanding of how work is normally done (Work-As-Normal) and what happened on the day itself (Work-As-Done).

We then build a simple timeline, having sufficient elements of Work-As-Done to build a picture of the incident, but primarily highlighting where the Work-As-Done related to the incident differed from the Work-As-Intended and/or Work-As-Normal. We will explore these gaps, or differences, in the next phase of the investigation.

As it relates to incident investigations, the Work-As-Intended line in Figure 3.2 represents the procedure or work instruction and the prehistoric view of safety was that if you followed that, you would not interact with the hazard and therefore not get hurt. The Work-As-Done line in Figure 3.2 represents what happened in the incident and the Work-As-Normal line is how the task is normally done by others. What is interesting to think about in Figure 3.2 is that the incident – the Work-As-Done line – comes from normal work. Up to a certain point in time, you can see work being done in a variety of ways – sometimes more safe and sometimes less safe – but we cannot tell whether it will end up in an incident (Work-As-Done), in innovation (above and beyond the Work-As-Intended line) or less safe (below the Work-As-Intended line).

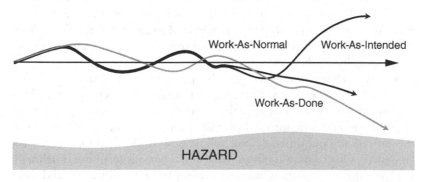

Figure 3.2 Work-As-Done, Work-As-Normal and Work-As-Intended

For your consideration:

Go out into the plant, take a few procedures with you and watch the world go by for a while. Get to understand whether Work-As-Normal = Work-As-Intended.

Determining Work-As-Done, Work-As-Normal and Work-As-Intended in the case of more detailed incident investigations

People have been creating timelines in relation to workplace incidents for many years. Timelines developed out of tools such as 'events and condition charting' and the need for people to understand the cause-and-effect nature of industrial accidents and incidents – or at least attempt to understand them. But methods and ideas are changing, and incident timelines now form the basis for a different way of thinking about incidents and their contributory causes.

When creating timelines as part of a detailed investigation, and indeed when people undertake interviews for this level of investigation, they must have an awareness of the concepts of Work-As-Done, Work-As-Normal and Work-As-Intended. Moreover, they need to understand that the gaps between Work-As-Done, Work-As-Normal and Work-As-Intended are the main drivers for the remainder of the investigation work.

This is why, when we are having conversations or carrying out interviews as part of the investigation, we need to talk not only with those directly involved or who saw what happened, but also to others who normally do the work.

Let's say an incident has occurred involving an electrician who received an electric shock from a live terminal in a distribution board during an electrical testing process. The conversation with the electrician who got the shock should initially focus predominantly on how they *normally* do this work – what normally happens. We need to also talk with electricians from other shifts or areas who do similar sorts of work, and establish how they normally do the work.

Yes, we are interested in what the procedure says, but we are also extremely interested in exploring the differences between how the electrician did the task on the day of the incident (Work-As-Done), how they and other electricians normally do this task (Work-As-Normal) and how the procedures and other systems tell us how to do the task (Work-As-Intended). Our take-aways from these conversations form the timeline.

Once the investigation team has completed the PEEPO and collected the information they said they would (including all relevant

Work-As-Intended documents), they focus on building the Work-As-Done and Work-As-Normal timelines by going through the data that has been gathered as well as the information from interviews.

Often, the way a specific action was done on the day of the incident matches the way that the work teams normally do that task.

Here is a simple example:

- How we normally do the work: "Take Fives are always completed prior to starting the task."
- Work-As-Done during the incident: "The operator completed a Take Five."

(For those of you not aware of the concept, Take Fives are a process used in many industries that attempt to get the operator, maintainer or whatever to take a few minutes to think through the task they are about to do and to think about what could go wrong and what they need to do to make sure it does not go wrong.) This example shows there was no gap between Work-As-Done and Work-As-Normal. This is not to say that this aligns with the Work-As-Intended, which is what the procedures and systems require. That is the next step.

There are two approaches to the actual building of the timelines and the choice is completely yours as to which you prefer. I suggest that you try them both and then make a call as to which you like better. I have seen both used within the same organization so I suggest you do not get too hung up about it all. The first method I will describe involves the creation of the Work-As-Done and Work-As-Normal timelines first and then building the Work-As-Intended timeline where it makes sense in relation to what you are seeing in the other components of the timeline. So, to do this, the team continues to slowly build up the timeline of what happened on the day of the incident and checks whether it matches the way that each of those tasks are normally done. Once this is complete, the investigation team moves on to examine the Work-As-Intended material to see if there are any gaps between Work-As-Done, Work-As-Normal and Work-As-Intended.

This activity should also endeavour to find out if any elements of Work-As-Intended are missing from the other timelines. This could indicate a problem with either the Work-As-Intended or the behaviour in the field.

The second method is the other way around. You first build the Work-As-Intended timeline and then explore where there is alignment and where there are gaps between Work-As-Done, Work-As Normal and Work-As-Intended. This method works well when your organization has a strong set of processes and systems that drive task assignment and monitoring

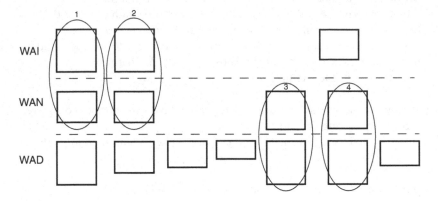

Figure 3.3 A completed timeline

or are very checklist-driven. The method would work well in cockpits and healthcare industries where checklists and protocols are common. The intent is still to explore any gaps between how the work was done on the day, how the work is normally done and how it is intended to be done.

Both of these processes are extremely simple in practice. In addition, I have found this way of creating timelines really helps to minimize any blame culture that may have crept into the investigation processes over time. A completed timeline could look like Figure 3.3.

For your consideration:

Spend some time with your people in the field, in the ward or on the plant over the next few weeks with the intent of trying to find out how the work is actually done, not just how the procedure or THA or standard thinks is the way the work should be done.

Exploration of the gaps between Work-As-Done, Work-As-Normal and Work-As-Intended

Once an investigation team has identified any gaps between Work-As-Done, Work-As-Normal and Work-As-Intended, they need to think about *why* those gaps exist. The topics described in this section, and in more detail in Chapter 4, can be used as a starting point to explore key drivers. But do not stop there – rather, use them as a starting point for conversations within the incident investigation team. Use the information and data that you've gathered up to this point and take advantage of the brains in the team. This is where the power of diversity in your investigation team can really be harnessed. The process is the same when undertaking a simple Outcome Analysis as it is for when you undertake a more detailed incident investigation up to and including significant and fatal incident investigations.

The exploration of these gaps has historically been carried out with a '5-whys' approach, which is a cross-examination technique used to determine the root cause of a problem by repeatedly asking questions starting with 'Why?' while building on the previous question.

But I actually prefer to frame the 5-whys questions as 'Hows & Whys', which I think is easier to handle and more powerful. I have removed the '5' from '5-whys' as it seems to cause confusion for some. I have seen many people get frustrated when they can get only four whys and their managers tell them they need five whys, or when they have got to five whys and have not yet quite got to where they hoped to get and want to add some more whys. This last problem can be made worse by well-meaning safety people who create spreadsheets with only five whys in it and no space for more. Asking "How did this come about?" instead of "Why did this happen?" can also open up another level of conversation. Moreover, it is less accusative.

Let's say an incident occurs where a maintainer used an old THA when actually the requirement is for a THA to be freshly written each time it is used. The task has changed since the original THA was created, one step in the process was missed and the maintainer was injured as a result. During the investigation it was determined that the way the work was normally done (Work-As-Normal) matched the Work-As-Intended insofar as the team normally used new THAs, but this individual, the maintainer who was injured, was the only employee who used an old THA. This meant there was a difference between Work-As-Done and Work-As-Intended, and also between Work-As-Done and Work-As-Normal.

The investigation could have stopped there with some "name, shame, blame and re-train" – as Todd Conklin so eloquently puts it – or human resources department involvement, to make sure the maintainer followed the rules next time around.

Using a Hows & Whys process, however, resulted in the following questions and answers:

Q. How did we end up with a maintainer using an old, off-the-shelf THA?

A. Because the maintainer thought the procedure allowed him to use an old THA.

> Q. How did the maintainer not know that the requirement to use a new THA was in the procedure?
>
> A. Because the procedure had changed twelve months ago and he was away on leave for six months and was not told of the change when he got back from leave.
>
> Q. How did we miss telling the maintainer about procedural changes when he returned from his long leave?
>
> A. Because the Management of Change process does not require that we identify those away from the workplace for extended periods of time, nor make sure they are aware of the managed change upon their return.

As you can see from this example, the Hows & Whys process does not always have to yield five questions and answers.

Once the Hows & Whys activity has been completed for each of the areas where gaps exist between any of Work-As-Done, Work-As-Normal and Work-As-Intended, we move to the creation of SMARTS actions or to an Incident Cause Analysis Method (ICAM) if that is what you are doing (see Appendix B).

Make sure you have asked enough questions and delved deeply enough during the Hows & Whys to get to a point where you are clearly looking at a high level, organizational explanation for the identified gap between Work-As-Done, Work-As-Normal and/or Work-As-Intended. This should be a much less formalized process for simpler incident investigations using Outcome Analyses than for more detailed incident investigations.

The beauty of thinking about what is driving any observable gaps between Work-As-Done, Work-As-Normal and Work-As-Intended is that it applies just as well before we have an incident as it does after an incident. I have been greatly inspired by Todd Conklin in his book *Pre-Accident Investigations*. After reading it, hearing him speak in a workshop and listening to his podcasts, I started to view the conversations we have before an incident as the same as the ones we have afterwards.

Okay. Back on topic. Below is a list of some of the common explanations for gaps between Work-As-Done, Work-As-Normal and Work-As-Intended. I encourage you to think about them as you explore your workplace both before and after an incident. There is a lot more detail provided in Chapter 4.

I do not want you to consider the following as a definitive list of causes or contributory factors. They are simply useful topics to understand and have in the back of your mind as you explore what happened in the workplace incident and why.

When I first started using this list I found that I tended to limit my thinking to what was in the list. This was a mistake. I have since learned to review this material before the investigation and keep it, along with an open mind, as a list of things to think about, explore and see if they are relevant or not. Below is a summary of the topics that I find useful to think about. There is much more detail on each to be found in Chapter 4 of this book. Chapter 4 also goes into more detail with respect to who and where these topics have come from.

Task complexity, procedural complexity and adequacy, or situational complexity

Humans are generally capable of doing more than one thing at a time, but only if those additional tasks are easy and understandable. If things start to get complicated or there is too much complexity, it becomes a high possibility that we lose focus, become overwhelmed and falter.

Sometimes, we try to put everything into a procedure. What can result is a procedure, or set of procedures, that can be neither clearly understood nor followed.

Resilience and resilience engineering

Resilience is often described as the ability to bounce back, to accommodate 'unexpected' change and to absorb uncertainties without falling apart.

There are four abilities or capabilities that describe resilience. These are the ability to respond to events, the ability to monitor ongoing developments, the ability to anticipate future threats and the ability to learn from past failures.

Risk intelligence, risk identification and risk management

Risk intelligence is the ability to estimate probabilities and likelihood accurately. An example could be that of understanding what the probability is of my actions leading to a car accident or a workplace incident. Another is that of understanding what the likelihood is that some piece of information we have just come across is actually true.

We often need to make educated guesses about such things, but fifty years of research in the psychology of judgement and decision-making show that most people are not very good at doing so. The more we force imprudent procedures on our people, the more we put up signs and mandate specific methods, the less risk intelligent they become.

Drift (procedural or practical drift)

Basically, drift explores whether the way we do the task today has changed slowly over a period of time. If it has, we need to find out whether the change, or the drift, has led to a higher level of risk in the outcome of the incident being investigated.

Internal decision- and sense-making

What was going on in the minds of the individuals involved at the time of the incident? How did the world look to them? How were they making sense of their surroundings? What led to the decision they made 'in the moment'? What was meaningful in what they saw?

Intense task focus

Intense task focus is all about humans making erroneous assessments and then being blind to other options or assessments. Such an approach can lead to an incorrect action, or indeed no action being taken at all.

Answering a different question – i.e. doing not what was asked, even if it is perceived as an easier task

If given an option, we tend to follow the path that requires the least effort. We often answer questions without much scrutiny as to whether the answer is truly appropriate, or we answer an easier question without noticing we have done so. Alternatively, we attempt to answer the question with an answer that seems intuitively to be correct, as it is easier to do so than to stop and think about it. A common area related to 'answering a different question' within incidents is in relation to task allocation by a supervisor.

What-You-See-Is-All-There-Is and Plan Continuation

What-You-See-Is-All-There-Is was coined by Daniel Kahneman and is one of those cognitive biases that we all experience. We assume, quite subconsciously, that what we see is all that we need to see, particularly when we are mapping out the scenario that could lead to a certain, or expected, outcome. Also, once a person has a plan in place, they start to follow that plan and tend not to change or stop the work, even when small signs emerge indicating they should stop and reconsider their approach.

Shared space as it relates to safe workspaces

'Shared space' is a way of thinking derived from a traffic-management philosophy but equally applies in any workplace. It originally involved the removal of traffic controls such as stop signs, traffic lights, speed limits, pedestrian crossings, barriers and gates, caution and warning signs, painted lines between different traffic users and so on. The idea is to increase the unease of road users and encourage mutual respect and communication – either direct or indirect, including eye contact and visual cues – in order for all road and intersection users to interact safely and effectively. Not only should we look out for too many signs in the workplace, but also think about whether they actually add value or not.

Effective 'core competency training' and 'awareness induction'

Inductions are all about raising awareness in the people exposed to the risks of the workplace so that they have cause to stop and think before barging off in a direction they may later regret. Core competency training is about making absolutely sure that the person being trained knows exactly what to do in their job. Moreover, they have proven they can do it through effective competency assessments. In relation to incident investigations, it is all about asking questions about the training; whether it is competency-based, a simple induction or some combination of the two. Do not make an assumption about competency when you hear or read that a person has been 'trained'.

Individual perspectives

People base all of their actions on their view of the world at that point in time and space. This might seem logical, but it is often overlooked when we are analysing the decision-making process that played a part in an incident.

If you are investigating an incident, then understanding the views and actions of the individual involved is critical – they have a different view of their world than you do, particularly as you only see it after an incident has happened (through the eyes of hindsight bias).

Systems of work and their interrelationships

To further understand a particular individual's assessments and subsequent actions, we can explore how the systems interacted with each other. Imagine an electrician carrying out some testing work in a confined space. He is working at height with a boilermaker cutting a pipe with an oxy-acetylene torch next to him. Consider how many procedures the electrician is expected to follow. How many systems are designed to give him directives? (E.g. working at height, hot work, permit to work, confined space and live electrical testing are a few that come to mind.) When an incident occurs, it is often the interaction of the systems that makes the difference, not just one system on its own.

It is all obvious when you know the outcome (hindsight bias)

Sidney Dekker, in *The Field Guide to Understanding 'Human Error'*, says "Hindsight changes how we look at past decision-making. It turns real, convoluted complexity into a simple linear story." Once a workplace incident has happened and we hear about it, we build this 'simple linear story' very quickly in our minds, usually completely at the subconscious level. Watch out for this.

Accountability and authority mismatch

These days there seems to be a significant industry push to hold people to account for their actions, particularly after something has gone wrong. Before jumping on board with this thinking, stop for a moment – and ask yourself a few questions: Did the people you are holding accountable have the authority to make decisions about their work? Did they have the capability and authority to carry out the work the way you believe it should be done?

Equipment, tools and plant design

One area that often gets forgotten during both simple Outcome Analyses and more detailed incident investigations is that of the equipment and tools we ask people to use and the design of the workspace we expect them to work in. Determining to what level the equipment, tools and plant design were optimal and created a workplace where it was possible to work safely to begin with is an essential component of any workplace incident investigation.

Task planning, assignment, acceptance and monitoring

To maximize the likelihood that a task will be undertaken effectively with the desired production and safety outcomes, some effort needs to go into setting it up for success. It needs to be understood and then planned in such a way as to take into consideration what is going on around the task, who is going to carry out the task, what tools and equipment are available, what procedures or other specific instructions need to be in play and what time restrictions may be appropriate. After the planning, we need to make sure both the supervisor and the worker carrying out the work agree on what needs to be done, why it needs to be done, what competencies the worker needs and what tools, equipment, methods, hazard controls and permits may be needed to carry out the work.

Once the task is under way, it is vital that there is a process in place to ensure that the work is being done as per the agreement and plan. So, in an investigation, there is ample opportunity to explore whether these things were all in place, what the quality and effectiveness of them was and whether there were any gaps. (Work-As-Done in the area of task planning, assignment, acceptance and monitoring compared to Work-As-Intended in that space.)

Leadership

A common element for both simple and more detailed incident investigations is the role leadership plays in setting up the individual or system prior to the unfolding of the incident. The conversations leaders have both before and after an incident are also very important in tracking any gaps that may have arisen between Work-As-Intended and Work-As-Done.

Other cognitive biases and heuristics

A heuristic is, roughly speaking, a rule of thumb which we all use every day to help us make decisions.

Biases are systematic errors and can be viewed as deviations from rational decision-making. Some of interest to us, and further explored in Chapter 4, include:

• availability bias;
• completeness bias;
• confirmation bias;
• control bias (illusion of control);
• escalation bias;
• framing effect;
• Fundamental Attribution Effect (error);
• Gambler's Fallacy;
• Neglect of Probability;
• outcome bias;
• Peltzman Effect (risk compensation); and
• planning fallacy.

The Efficiency–Thoroughness Trade-Off

Efficiency–Thoroughness Trade-off (ETTO) is the work of Eric Hollnagel and is described in great detail in his book of the same name. In virtually all we do at work and at play, we make choices that try to strike a balance between being efficient and being thorough. In all levels of workplace incident investigations it is worth trying to understand the balance between efficiency and thoroughness and what the ETTO balance actually was in relation to the activity, remembering that the ETTO balance can be at an individual level and also at an organizational level.

For your consideration:

Spend some time reading Chapter 4 and think about some of the science that goes behind the above topics.

In your current incident investigation process, how much effort goes into what lies behind the actions people take, as compared to simply the behaviour itself?

Where on the ETTO balance do your current incident investigations sit?

Build the story (Incident Pathway Statement)

At this point in time, we have a good understanding of Work-As-Done, Work-As-Normal and Work-As-Intended. We have explored 'how' and 'why' we ended up with the gaps between Work-As-Done, Work-As-Normal and Work-As-Intended. From this – and other information gathered earlier on in the piece – we have built our understanding of the incident.

Now it is time to build our story of the incident. The idea of describing the incident as a story is based on elements within *Safety Differently* by Sidney Dekker. In this, he talks about the need for multiple perspectives to describe complexity. He says "Truth, then, lies in diversity of explanations and narratives, not in singularity." In a similar vein, describing the incident and how it came about requires the use of narrative or narratives. Care needs to be taken to ensure the story told represents the various perspectives and views and does not strive for a single 'root cause' so often sought for in incident investigation reports. Telling the story is a powerful way of steering the incident investigation report reader away from this concept of a root cause. A root cause is a useful concept when we have a simple mechanical failure, or incident that is so simple as to not need an investigation, where cause and effect live happily together. However, for incidents that are more complex, simple Newtonian cause and effect and the search for a simple root cause is not useful at all. Many incidents encountered in a modern technical or healthcare situation are complex and so a story is a better method to describe the incident and how it came about.

So, we build a story. A story that can sit nicely at home in an executive summary of the incident investigation report, and be so logical that anyone can read it and gain a good sense of what happened and why. There may well be a number of stories involved in the incident, and these all need to be told, but they need to be consistent with the findings of the incident.

Here is an example to give you a sense of what a story might look and sound like for a reasonably detailed incident. The first section below sets the scene of the incident that the story is built on:

Incident

On 25 March, the concentrator and filter plant storm water handling system became stressed due to a high rainfall event. In order to control the water level of the retention pond to prevent it overflowing, a valve was required to be opened on an elevated pipe gantry.

An operator accessed a scaffold, which was in the area due to a recent maintenance shut, and then climbed off the scaffold to access and operate the valve. This was done without any fall arrest or fall prevention equipment or controls.

Physical findings

There was no physical barrier on the scaffold to prevent a person leaving the scaffold at height.

The scaffold tag indicated the scaffold was safe to access yet hand and knee rails were missing, potentially exposing operators or maintainers to a fall from height hazard.

What people did (derived from gaps between Work-As-Done, Work-As-Normal and Work-As-Intended)

The scaffolders left the scaffold (and the area) with the scaffold in an unsafe condition, yet the scaffold tag indicated it was safe to use.

The operator left the confines of the scaffold and accessed a pipe rack approximately 4 metres above the ground without using any fall arrest or fall prevention equipment.

The operator did not assess or discuss the task or situation prior to commencing the task (he did not ask what could go wrong or think about what to do if it did).

The supervisor gave an instruction to the operator to carry on with work, without having a discussion with respect to the hazards, hazard controls, required training and task steps.

Explanation of gaps between Work-As-Done, Work-As-Normal and Work-As-Intended

The Site Scaffold Procedure is vague with respect to when a scaffold tag must be removed or turned during dismantling of a scaffold or when the scaffold is not in direct control of the scaffolder.

Scaffolders or other scaffolding experts were not involved in the final ratification, or approval of the site scaffold procedure.

The site does not include any training or competencies associated with ensuring operators and maintainers have a sound understanding of resilience or risk intelligence.

The Corporate Safe Work Standard, which includes the requirements for how a supervisor is to assign tasks, was not rolled out beyond the general manager of the operation as the operation was waiting (for six months) for guidance and training material from the corporate office.

Explanations at an organizational factor level

The site process for the creation of operational procedures does not require task experts (such as scaffolders) to approve or ratify final versions of operating procedures.

An analysis of the operation's Training Needs Analysis reveals that the only required skills to carry out tasks are technical in nature. There is no mention of supporting skills such as resilience, risk intelligence, risk management, decision-making, fatality risk-related awareness (such as working at height), etc.

The corporate office does not have a process for the simultaneous issuing of guidance and training materials when it issues new, or amended standards and corporate procedures to the operation.

What are the stories contained in this incident?

Incident Pathway Statement:

As the corporate office does not have a process to ensure appropriate training and guidance material is issued with new or modified

Standards and Corporate Procedures, the site was left with a six-month-old standard that it did not roll out. A direct consequence of this was that a relatively new supervisor gave a set of instructions to an operator without ensuring the operator had the right training and competencies, was aware of the hazards and required hazard controls and knew exactly what the task entailed and why it was needed. The operator then carried out a task without taking into consideration what training he should have had, without identifying the risks and without the appropriate working-at-height protective systems.

In addition to these issues, the site's process to create operating procedures does not require technical expert sign-off. This meant the procedure was vague with respect to scaffold tag removal. When the scaffolders temporarily left the scaffold, an operator saw a scaffold tag and made the assumption that the scaffold was safe, when, in fact, it was not.

The final cog in this incident was that an operator was exposed to a working at height hazard, and he was not aware of the risk due to the fact that the Training Needs Analysis at the operation contained only the required technical skills to carry out tasks, not the supporting skills such as resilience, risk intelligence and management, decision-making, fatality risk-related awareness (such as working at height), etc.

The required skill in creating the Incident Pathway Statement is seeing the story build as you unfold the explanations for the gaps between Work-As-Done, Work-As-Normal and Work-As-Intended during your Hows & Whys step. If you are doing an ICAM (see Appendix B for a description of this technique), then it is simply a matter of converting the ICAM chart from a graphical representation into a few paragraphs that tell the story. The Incident Pathway Statement should easily hang together and help a reader who is unfamiliar with the details of the incident understand the investigation team's view of what happened and why. It should read like you are telling someone about the incident.

For your consideration:

What stories do you tell when describing incidents that have occurred in your business?

Next time you are asked to explain an incident to someone, try using a story instead of just the 'causes' and 'contributing factors'.

SMARTS actions

I often get asked which I prefer: a high-quality investigation with poor corrective actions or a poor-quality investigation with high-quality corrective actions. The answer is always a simple one – I say that I would go for high-quality actions any day. This is still true, but I believe also that the story, the learning that has come from the investigation, is just as important. Especially in relation to how well the story has been shared and learned from. For me, the corrective actions associated with a workplace incident investigation are the manifestation, or creation, of the investigation itself. They represent the incident's story, as discovered by the investigation team, which is why both the story and the actions are important. The actions embody what the future will look like after the dust has settled. In fact, corrective and preventive actions are what ensure that we do not have a repeat incident.

Corrective actions need to be easily executable, and should really only be tied to the reasons lying behind the gaps identified between Work-As-Done, Work-As-Normal and Work-As-Intended, keeping what we discussed in the 'explanations' section front of mind. In other words, from information gleaned during the Hows & Whys process.

It is important to remember that actions are things we want someone to do. They are work. If we remember this, it makes life a lot easier to create an action with SMARTS.

Okay, so what does SMARTS actually mean? I do not mean that these actions must be intelligent and therefore not be stupid (though that is certainly a plus!). SMARTS is an acronym:

S – Specific
M – Measurable
A – Achievable
R – Relevant
T – Time-bound
S – Sustainable

Let's take a moment and break these down individually.

Specific

An action needs to be specific if we want it to be understood and done as we plan it to be. The language should be succinct, and it must make sense to the person doing the task – i.e. not in any way confusing or vague. A good example would be something like:

Remove the ball valve on the entry line immediately prior to sump pump SP 106 in the beneficiation plant. Replace it with a gate valve. In selecting the gate valve, remember that when the valve is fully open the flow through the valve needs to match the flow rate of the ball valve.

A poor example would be: "Investigate the possibility of replacing the ball valve with a gate valve." This is not specific inasmuch as we have no clue which valve needs replacing.

Measurable

We need to know when the action is completed – and a good indicator of that is when we can see that specific changes have been made. "Investigate the possibility of changing out the ball valve for a gate valve" is not measurable. How can we tell when we have 'investigated the possibility' of something? Better wording could be: "Carry out a formal engineering study and issue a formal report concerning the feasibility of changing out the ball valve (on the entry line immediately prior to sump pump SP 106 in the beneficiation plant) with a gate valve."

Achievable

Do not try to boil the ocean or save the whales here. After all, we need to be able to pull the action off. It's easy to fall into the trap of setting too many aspirational goals, rather than actions we can actually achieve. I recall one particular case, which in essence suggested the actioner "improve the safety culture of the mine with a higher level of worker involvement". To me, this is not even setting work, but is a vague wish or theme for a larger set of work activities. The actions arising from an investigation need to be achievable.

Relevant

Team members should not add actions that are not directly relevant to the incident. I recall a fatality investigation where an action related to control of the underground magazine inventories ended up in a fatality investigation action list. The mine leadership team were so occupied with this action that they excluded others that played a more significant role in the fatality.

Time-bound

We never really know how busy people are. So always have a chat with the person you think should do the action before assigning it to them.

Not only can you then figure out if they are the right person for the job, but you will also be able to ask how long it will take them to do it. Simply assigning a task to someone without talking to them about it is fraught with danger – having had no input into the creation of the action, the person may not feel as keen to see it carried out as you may be. Even though we think the action is important, it may not be a priority for them. Particularly when other tasks, which they deem more important, are already taking up their time.

I have seen, for example, a two-week deadline given to an action that entailed modifying and rolling out a procedure. In my experience, such a time frame is more often than not unattainable. It is not possible to engage with the end users of the procedure, gather their input, make changes accordingly, get the revisions reviewed and approved and carry the new procedure through the document control system within two weeks – not forgetting we then have to make sure that all of those impacted by the changes across the shifts are aware of and competent in the new processes. We are simply setting someone up to fail if we put such a target in place.

Sustainable

One thing that often happens is investigation teams create actions that have no life beyond the immediate. Having a sustainable action means having one that will still exist in a year's time or longer. They are generally systems-based. They are not necessarily an addition to a procedure but embedded somehow in the way that we do work. It could be changing some training or induction material or process. An example of an action that is not sustainable is "send a message at the next round of safety talks to remind the workers to be more careful".

A word or two of caution for the newbie to incident investigations: watch out for actions that seem simple and common, but are actually wholly ineffective. Examples that come to mind include statements like: "Retrain those involved in the incident", "Retrain the work force in risk management" or "Reinforce the importance of safety to the workforce".

With respect to the first two examples, it has become commonplace over the years to use 'training' as a corrective action. Although it appears easy, there are a couple of reasons why it is usually useless. One is that the person at the centre of the investigation is by now fully aware of their 'failing' and certainly does not need to sit through another training session on the topic. The second is that training everybody else will just annoy them and cause frustration in the workplace. If the training was not effective the first time, why should it be any different this time? Keeping this in mind, the only time training should rate a mention in a list of corrective actions is if the investigation has identified problems with the training itself. The action would then be about fixing the training, not automatically repeating it and expecting a different outcome. The third example of an ineffective action is also, sadly, very common. I often see actions that are motherhood statements and not actions at all. These sorts of corrective actions should get picked up when exploring whether the action is measurable, as part of the SMARTS stage, but they often slip through.

The fundamental rules for assigning corrective actions – which must be followed in every case – are to make sure the person is aware of the action, agrees that they are the best person accountable for its completion and understands the context and purpose of the corrective action. We too often see actions fail because they are assigned to the wrong person – someone who is not interested in the action and has no context of why the action needs doing in the first place.

One more thing: avoid human resources actions in a safety incident investigation. Most organizations have models for 'Just Culture' or 'Fair Play' and processes designed to apportion blame – ranging from culpable individual action to organizational fault. Generally, these processes are neither just nor fair. They are inconsistently applied across departments and used to justify written warnings and sackings. They are not about accountability at all. I suggest a good reading of Sidney Dekker's *Just Culture* will help cure any of you who disagree with this paragraph.

For your consideration:

Review a handful of recent incident investigation reports and see how many of the corrective actions are SMARTS.

Reports

Each operation and company will have its own reporting requirements. The biggest learning I can share with you in this space is to challenge what you have and make it as simple as you can, but not too simple.

So, what should be in a report? A great place to start thinking about an answer to the question is to ask your leaders about the purpose of the report. Is it to share findings, learn something, help senior leaders understand the incident, simply capture the outcome of the investigation or some mixture of these? The reason this question is important is that, as you may well have experienced in your own business, incident investigation report templates tend to grow over time. People want an additional statistic, or bit of information added because they think it might be important or useful. Over time, drift creeps in and we end up with a twenty-page report instead of a five-page report. We see a similar trend in procedures over time. One way of bucking this trend is to challenge the senior leadership teams about why the form looks like it does. Making it simple will often result in better-quality reports as the incident investigation team can focus on the important things and not the fluff that someone thinks they want to see.

For me, a model investigation report for a detailed incident contains the following, as a maximum:

- Incident details: when, where, what and a one-paragraph overview of the incident. This should not attempt to explain how the outcome came about but is purely a description of the incident.
- Timelines and identified gaps or differences between Work-As-Done, Work-As-Normal and Work-As-Intended: I use a word table for this with the gaps and differences highlighted as I think they work better than graphics or spreadsheets for this work.
- Hows & Whys: including the questions and the answers.
- The Incident Pathway Statement (story): this is really an executive summary of the investigation.
- The ICAM chart/list (if you have done an ICAM – see Appendix B): either a graphic version or a list. This needs to include all of the absent/failed defences, individual/team actions, task/environmental conditions and organizational factors.
- Key learnings: this should be one or two sentences that really capture the most important elements and thought provokers that came from the incident and subsequent investigation.
- Actions: should all be SMARTS, of course.

The best reports I have seen for simple Outcome Analyses are split into three sections. The first part is an overview of the event – including the what, where and when. This is followed with a simple timeline showing the differences between Work-As-Done, Work-As-Normal and Work-As-Intended only (a complete timeline should not be attempted here; leave that for the detailed incident investigations). Include a summary of the gaps identified. A simple story about the incident should also be included – one that is so logical that anyone can read it and gain a good sense of what happened and why. There may well be a number of stories involved in the incident, but they need to be consistent with the findings of the incident. The third section should contain a couple of suggestive actions, which should be undertaken to close those gaps.

As for sharing, there is nothing more useless than going to all the trouble of carrying out a detailed incident investigation, coming up with some actions and then not sharing the story with your organization. This is where the Incident Pathway Statement comes so much into play. The whole idea of the Incident Pathway Statement is to tell the story of the incident to others. If it is well written, in a conversational style, it will lend itself to sharing. If others understand what was going on in the incident in a way that gels with them, the learning will be real and they will remember it as they come across similar situations into the future.

For your consideration:

Is your reporting pro forma full of 'nice-to-haves' that nobody looks at, or does it only contain the information that is necessary and useful to the reader?

Is your reporting system accessible and easy to use?

Do your reports differentiate themselves between simple and more detailed incidents and their investigations?

How well do you share the learnings from an incident investigation?

4 The technical and scientific stuff

This chapter is designed for those of you who seek more details lying behind the concepts used in the process described in the other chapters of this book. It should be read along with the Bibliography. I have simply used the names of the authors of material rather than a formal referencing process here as this is not intended as a technical reference but as an enticer for you to seek more information. The books, papers and comments in the Bibliography should act as a first pass for getting details beyond that covered in this chapter. My goal is to pique your interest to learn more about the concepts that lie behind both the Outcome Analysis and more detailed incident investigation processes. Getting a sound understanding of the topics and ideas covered in this chapter of the book will greatly enhance your ability to understand what lies behind some of the human behaviours you see in workplace incidents and to help you understand what is driving worker activities more generally. Enjoy.

Task complexity, procedural complexity and adequacy and situational complexity

Humans are generally capable of doing more than one thing at a time, but only if the additional tasks we ask of them are easy to do and readily understandable. If things start to get complicated, or if there is too much complexity going on, it becomes a high possibility that we lose focus, become overwhelmed and falter.

As a result of drift, actions from workplace incident investigations and system audits, we sometimes end up putting more and more information and work requirements into a procedure. What can result is a procedure, or set of procedures, that can be neither clearly understood nor easily followed. It is important to remember that we can be greatly affected by what is going on around us in our workplaces; the more complexity that's involved, the higher the level of risk of not being able to do what is required.

Understanding the level of complexity and managing it is thus vital to the safe completion of tasks. Complex and complicated actually mean different things. Many procedures are simply complicated. I once heard Todd Conklin describe 'complicated' during a workshop using the following analogy: "Building a nuclear submarine is complicated. If you have the right parts, the right skills to put them together, the right tools and the right instruction manual, it is possible. Difficult, but possible."

He went on to say that 'complex' on the other hand is about a system that is not completely knowable. Where inputs do not always yield the outcomes you expect, or where systems interact with each other in ways that are unexpected or unknowable. "Raising a child is complex," Todd said. Increasingly, our socio-technical processes in our plants, operations and hospitals are complex, in addition to being complicated. Everything interacts with everything else. Sidney Dekker has a similar view. In *Patient Safety* he says that complicated systems are ultimately knowable and that complex systems, in contrast, are never fully knowable.

If you are working with a complex or unruly technology, having strict procedures and strict procedural compliance expectations is fraught with danger. If you attempt to control a complex process with procedures, the resultant procedures themselves will become so complicated that they may also become complex. Complex procedures do not work.

Many people view the healthcare industry as simply complicated, rather than complex, which it clearly is. This mistake is often also made within sections of other industries. Even the apparently simple process of mining has elements and parts of the whole that are complex, and yet they are viewed as complicated and attempts are made to excessively proceduralize the work. In both the healthcare and elements of the minerals-extraction industries, amongst many others, the result is procedures that people do not, or in fact often cannot, follow. And then subsequent witch hunts that masquerade as incident investigations follow when things go wrong.

Determining whether a task, procedure or situation is complex is a subjective activity. We need to see if the procedural or situational requirements exceed the capacity of the person doing the task. We also need to understand in what way those involved made sense of the world, the task requirements and whether these matched the world-view that the creator of the procedure, situation or task had.

A determination of the complexity of a procedure, task or situation requires a non-hindsight-biased analysis and this is not always easy. When looking into the level of complexity, think about what level of adaptive learning is required to get the job done. Also explore if the level of adaptive capacity of those involved in carrying out the task actually matches the level of complexity.

There is a common approach across much of industry at the moment to strive for simplicity in systems and procedures. As an investigation is progressing, it can be valuable to explore the balance between simplicity and complexity. Oversimplicity can cause just as much pain as complexity and complicatedness. There is also a balance between underproceduralization and overproceduralization to consider. In the words of Bieder and Bourrier in *Trapping Safety into Rules*, "There is no doubt that proceduralization and documented activities have in the past brought constant progress, avoided recurrent mistakes and allowed for 'best' practice to be adopted. Yet, it seems that the exclusive and intensive use of procedures today is in fact a threat to progress in safety." I feel that this drive to consider the procedure as king is more than just a threat to progress in safety. It is a threat to safety on a day-to-day basis.

The main point of this section is to alert the investigation team or the investigation leader to keep a close eye on the complexity and usefulness of the systems we ask people, or expect people, to follow as well as the situations we put them in as they do their work.

For your consideration:

Read through the procedures and forms that make up the Work-As-Intended for work being done in your workplace and determine how easy they are to follow correctly, or how easy they are to follow incorrectly.

While watching work being done, or talking about it, get a sense of whether the task is easy to do.

While watching work being done, or by talking about it, get a sense of whether it is easier to get the job done by taking shortcuts rather than following the rules.

Check out a couple of procedures over the next week or so. Ask about when the procedures of interest were last formally reviewed, and whether the process took into consideration the purpose of the document and whether it was written for the user, or whether it was written to satisfy some system requirement.

How well is your workplace configured? Do any of the structures create complexity and difficulty in getting the job done?

Resilience and resilience engineering

As we explore the differences between Work-As-Done, Work-As-Normal and Work-As-Intended, we cannot possibly leave out resilience, or resilience engineering as it is mainly referred to as in the works of Erik Hollnagel.[1] Resilience is often described as the ability to bounce back, to accommodate 'unexpected' change and to absorb uncertainties without falling apart.

We know that workplace incidents come from normal work. The point here is that we need to adapt to the changing environment in which we find ourselves as we undertake work. This is especially true in a complex and highly linked system, and one where we cannot adapt sufficiently, or in the right direction. It is often when we end up with an unexpected outcome – an incident. This is where resilience plays a major role.

According to Hollnagel, "it is both easier and more effective to increase safety by improving the number of things that go right, than reducing the number of things that go wrong". Resilience is one of those things that we can set up that will greatly assist in getting things right. Resilience or its absence is something we should always check for when undertaking any level of workplace incident investigation.

There are four abilities or capabilities that describe resilience. These are:

- the ability to respond to events;
- the ability to monitor ongoing developments;
- the ability to anticipate future threats; and
- the ability to learn from past failures.

We can have a direct and effective impact on the resilience of our people and our systems. Having conversations and setting up our systems, procedures and our expectations to include resilience will make a huge difference to our safety outcomes. The topic of resilience is a very powerful conversation starter when exploring what has led to any observed differences between Work-As-Done, Work-As-Normal and Work-As-Intended. This is just as true when investigating an incident as it is on a day-to-day basis.

If we are looking at a procedure, work instruction, THA or having a conversation with someone before or after an incident, we should include questions to see if resilience played a part. We need to find out the extent to which the people and systems involved in the incident were resilient. That should emerge not only from the written documentation that surrounds the incident, but also from conversations. I can recall many cases where I was shown a THA, along with the relevant procedures and work instructions during an incident investigation. All of these documents had been really well written; they pointed to the particular part of the task that may cause the worker grief, told them to watch out for certain indicators when things might start to go wrong and told them what to do to make sure the incipient incident did not manifest. These are all good traits of a resilient system.

In other cases, including in fatality investigations that I have facilitated, however, the worker has had no idea of what was in the procedure – so it did not matter whether the documentation was resilient or not. If the worker is not knowledgeable of the documentation, they are not guided by what is in it and hence may well not demonstrate much resilience themselves; they may have different ideas about which parts of the job could be a problem, and therefore may not have an adequate plan in place should things start to go pear-shaped.

A good question to ask is whether they truly understand which particular tasks within their job that day could cause them grief, and what they plan to do about it.

In summary, during both a simple incident investigation (Outcome Analysis) and a more detailed incident investigation, seek to understand how well the individuals involved understood, before the incident, what could have gone wrong. Did they also have a plan should it have gone wrong – and to what extent did the plan work? Try to gain a sense of how they normally keep an eye on things that may become a threat in the near future.

Much resilience can be created prior to work commencing, while the tasks are planned and conversations are held. As a work team pulls together a THA, for example, they can discuss what could go wrong, what indicators they should look out for that would tell them things were about to go wrong, and what they need to do if it starts to go wrong. This is building resilience into the job preparation.

In many ways anticipation is the cornerstone of resilience. It is the ability to think about what could happen, and then it is all about the adaptive capacity of the individuals concerned and the systems in which they work.

Helping people improve their judgement of the likelihood of outcomes and their assessment of the risks associated with following, or not following, procedures and guidance requires risk intelligence – the next topic.

For your consideration:

When you are in the field, plant or ward before an incident during a normal day, ask some questions that could help you understand how resilient the team is. For example:

- In the preparation of a Take Five or THA, what level of thought was put into what could go wrong?
- Which specific parts of a task do the team or individuals need to stay vigilant around?
- How best does the team prepare to respond to any expected disruptions?
- What does the individual or work team do if something unexpected happens?

Risk intelligence, risk identification and risk management

The way I am using the term 'risk intelligence' is taken from Dylan Evans and his book by the same name – well worth a read. Risk intelligence is the ability to estimate probabilities and likelihoods accurately. An example could be my level of understanding the probability that my actions could lead to a car accident, or a workplace incident. Another is understanding what the likelihood is that some piece of information we have just come across is actually true.

We often need to make educated guesses about such things, but fifty years of research in the psychology of judgement and decision-making show that most people are not very good at doing this. Many people, for example, tend to overestimate their chances of winning the lottery, while they underestimate the probability that they will suffer from cancer or a heart attack at some point in their life.

At the heart of risk intelligence lies the ability to gauge the limits of your own knowledge – to be cautious when you don't know too much, and to be confident when, by contrast, you know a lot.

Being able to understand the risk associated with an activity is vital to controlling the risk and completing the task in a safe and effective manner. It is just as important to understand the likelihood of an event turning out as planned as it is to understand the risk of an event not going to plan, or having an unexpected outcome.

In essence, risk intelligence is all about having the right degree of certainty to make sound decisions. The more we force imprudent procedures on our people, the more we put up signs and mandate specific methods, the less risk intelligent they become. We need to help them learn how to think again.

Risk intelligence is not the same as risk appetite, nor is it akin to other 'risk-isms' such as risk perception, risk loving, risk hating, risk avoidance, risk management, risk judgements, risk assessment, risk estimates, risk abatement, risk attitude or risk neutrality. In fact, it is all about the individual and their ability to judge and to know the limits of their own knowledge.

It is possible to help people improve their risk intelligence by providing feedback following a risk judgement. You could create a process where the worker is required to assess the level of risk associated with their work prior to the task and then carry out a task post-mortem after they finish the task. That way, they can assess how accurate their pre-task assessment was.

During one of his informative pre-accident podcasts, Todd Conklin referenced a set of questions for this purpose, which I think work wonders in this space:

- What went well?
- What did not go well?
- What hazards did we find (with particular focus on those that we did not expect)?
- What surprised us?

Instilling this sort of post-mortem activity as a habit will improve the risk intelligence of those doing the activity. They will also tend to do more efficient THAs, have a much better sense of the risk associated with a task and therefore create safe work more often. This touches on the topic of risk identification.

It is often illuminating to touch base with an individual after an incident, to see if they thought the outcome was possible, and if so, how much attention they gave the risk before the incident.

So, how do we make sure our people know they are creating safe work through their choices and their risk intelligence and risk assessments? One way is by being there as they do their normal day-to-day work, when there have not yet been any incidents. We can then explore the differences between Work-As-Done, Work-As-Normal and Work-As-Intended as work is being done.

We have covered risk intelligence in sufficient depth for now. Let's look at risk identification and risk management a bit more. In order to control or otherwise manage risk, we need to be able to identify risk. There is no doubt in my mind that this is a skill that can be learned. It is also possible to determine through conversation the level of skill the individual has around the topic of risk.

Paul Slovic puts the idea of risk very well in the title of his book *The Feeling of Risk*. How we feel about an issue has an enormous impact on our perception of the level of risk associated with the issue. He goes on to describe how we are not rational decision-makers and that risk is assessed not from a technical analysis using logic, statistics or decision theory, but it is rather driven by heuristics such as the availability heuristic and the representativeness and recency heuristics. I am reminded about Donald Rumsfeld's comments about what we know and what we don't know: "There are known knowns. These are things we know that we know. There are known unknowns. That is to say, there are things that we know we don't know. But there are also unknown unknowns. There are things we don't know we don't know." This is actually a very clever saying, even though it was lambasted at the time. It is especially relevant when we talk about risk inasmuch as it hits the mark in terms of what hazards and their associated risks are considered or not considered as a workplace incident develops. It is also a great conversation starter during the interview process.

An important aspect of risk management related to the study of workplace incidents lies with what is often called 'material', 'catastrophic' or 'fatality' risk management. A material risk is one where the maximum foreseeable loss is a single fatality or equivalent loss. All material risk frameworks that I have seen have 'critical' controls. These are risk controls that relate to specific material risks and are those controls that must remain fully effective for the material risk to be adequately managed.

As we explore the gaps between Work-As-Done, Work-As-Normal and Work-As-Intended, it is worth examining if any part of the Work-As-Intended includes such critical controls. This is important, not only with respect to the work being carried out, but also with respect to the systems that check and ensure the critical controls are in place and run efficiently. As a reminder, critical controls are those controls that relate to fatal and material risks put in place that must work each and every time a task is undertaken. In the case of critical controls associated with material or fatal risk, the risk identification process is partly taken away from the worker. This is a two-edged sword and the worker should still be encouraged to think about what other risks have raised their heads and not just the critical ones. Before risks can be managed or controlled they need to be identified by someone who is risk intelligent.

For your consideration:

How well did your organization prepare your front-line people and those involved in the incident to handle problems, assess risk and understand what the various likelihoods of their actions are?

When you are in an incident investigation or when you are in the field looking at the quality of THAs, do you challenge the team with respect to how they came up with their risk assessments?

Have you checked how well your organization highlights and focusses on the 'critical controls' of 'fatal risks' and 'material risks'?

Explore whether your induction and training processes aid your people in risk intelligence.

Drift (procedural or practical drift)

Basically, drift explores whether the way we do the task today has changed slowly over a period of time. If it has, we need to find out whether the change, or the drift, has led to a higher level of risk associated with the outcome of the incident being investigated. Scott Snook, in his great book *Friendly Fire: The Accidental Shootdown of US Black Hawks over Northern Iraq*, describes what he calls Practical Drift as "the slow steady uncoupling of local practice from written procedure". This is exactly the same concept as Dekker talks extensively about in *Drift into Failure: From Hunting Broken Components to Understanding Complex Systems*.

Drift is ubiquitous. It is present at work and at home. Think about the loss of the Space Shuttle Columbia on 1 February 2003. The official incident review found that a piece of foam insulation from the external tank had fallen onto the left wing of the shuttle and damaged the thermal protection system tiles. Drift played a significant part in this turn of events – particularly related to how NASA viewed foam loss and debris impact to the shuttle. Investigators found that when procedures were first introduced, maintainers repairing the foam insulation were required to report each damage event, which were regarded as safety events at the time. Over the following years, however, they shifted from being a flight safety issue to a maintenance issue. As such reports became rather common, and thus unremarkable, they often went unreported and hence there was no real understanding of the condition of the foam under the repairs. Also, the fact that the foam loss events had occurred regularly and changed over time from a real issue to 'normal'. The technical cause of the ultimate disaster was a large debris strike to the orbiter's wing from foam that had broken off the left bipod ramp that attached the shuttle to its large external liquid-fuel tank. In sixty-five of the seventy launches, foam debris had been seen so this was not a new or unexpected phenomenon. This is drift. You only have to pick up a procedure in your workplace that is a few years old and go into the field, the lab or the ward and watch how the work is actually getting done and then talk to people to see drift in action. You will hear things like "Yep, we used to do it that way, but now we ..."

For your consideration:

Look closely at procedures relating to work that is being done today. Have we changed the way we do the task to the detriment of safety?

Talk to people in your workplace about what changes they have seen in the way they do a task. Has it changed over the years?

Next time you are out and about in your plant, in the mine or on the ward in a hospital, ask a few people about drift and what changes they have seen over the years in how "work is done around here". Such an exercise can bring up a raft of new information worth considering by both the work crew and also you, as a manager or supervisor.

Internal decision- and sense-making

What was going on in the mind of the individuals involved at the time of the incident? How did the world look to them? How were they making sense of their surroundings? What led to the decision they made 'in the moment'? What was meaningful in what they saw? What did the situation 'mean' to those involved and present at the time? Was the sense-making of those directly involved in the incident the same as, or similar to, what we see now with the powerful 'benefit' of hindsight?

These questions, along with many more, spring to mind when starting to think about sense-making in the workplace.

There are many definitions of sense-making in the literature. I like one from Sally Maitlis and Marlys Christianson in their paper *Sensemaking in Organizations: Taking Stock and Moving Forward*. They describe sense-making as "The process through which people work to understand issues and events that are novel, ambiguous, confusing, or in some other way violate expectations." How we see the world has a direct and powerful impact on how we make decisions within that world. Further, Maitlis and Christianson go on to suggest that sense-making is an important process for learning. This puts it very much into the arena of resilience and risk intelligence also.

Barry and Meisiek, in their article *Seeing More and Seeing Differently: Sensemaking, Mindfulness and Their Workarts*, quote Weick to define collective mindfulness as "the capacity of groups and individuals to be acutely aware of significant details, to notice errors in the making, and to have the shared expertise and freedom to act on what they notice". This has big implications in the normalization of deviance, where we often do not see the problems as they are created and then, when nothing goes wrong, perpetuate the error again and again. Maitlis and Christianson also use an example we have already touched on. Instances of foam shedding from NASA space shuttles were reclassified over a long period of time from an "in-flight anomaly" to an "acceptable risk" that was not deemed to be a flight safety issue that would result in a disaster. This normalization of deviance is a classic example of sensemaking that in hindsight was not all that accurate an assessment of a situation. As you may see, this could be viewed as a driver of procedural drift also.

Asking questions of those involved in workplace incidents along with those involved in the various decisions and actions that may have preceded the incident about sense-making is time well spent during an investigation regardless of the level or complexity of the incident and its investigation. When you do this, remember that the sense-making you are applying in hindsight will in all probability be very different from the sense-making undertaken by those involved at the time of the incident. This is especially true as a result of a paradox that does nothing to promote 'good' sense-making as an incident unfolds; on the one hand, hazardous and rapidly unfolding situations are difficult to comprehend, so people want to gather more information in order to determine the most appropriate action. On the other hand, the demands of the situation often require them to take action with incomplete information.

For your consideration:

When you are walking around in your ward, unit, plant or mine, ask people to stop, take a break and look around their workplaces. What can they see? Was there anything that they previously did not know was there?

Are you surprised during an investigation, when someone says, "No, I did not see that?" You should not be.

Intense task focus

Also called cognitive fixation, intense task focus is all about humans making erroneous assessments and then being blind to other options or assessments. Such an approach can lead to an incorrect action, or indeed no action being taken at all.

You should explore whether intense task focus played a role in the event when exploring potential gaps between Work-As-Done, Work-As-Normal and Work-As-Intended. People also do not want, or maybe cannot even hear, more information that might spoil their story (What-You-See-Is-All-There-Is – see section below with the same title). You can become blind to what is in front of you.

This phenomenon is described in great detail in *The Invisible Gorilla* by Christopher Chabris and Daniel Simons. Go to www.theinvisiblegorilla. com to see a really powerful example regarding the number of basketball passes between a team, alongside many other examples.

The main point with respect to intense task focus is not to be surprised when someone tells you that they did not see something that you feel, with the benefit of hindsight, should have been very obvious at the time. Intense task focus can also manifest as people tend not to be able to see things that they do not expect to see. In a classic video of Chabris and Simons', a stranger is asked for direction advice. As the stranger is studying a piece of paper given to him by the actor, two workmen walk between them carrying an opaque door. As the door passes the stranger, the person seeking help from the stranger swaps out with one of the tradesmen so that when the door has passed, the stranger is now facing a different person. About 50% of people subjected to this experiment do not notice that the person has changed; it is not something they would expect and so therefore they do not see it. This occurs in work situations all the time and is worthy of your consideration as you attempt to solve the puzzle of the incident.

For your consideration:

Show your team the Invisible Gorilla video at www.theinvisiblegorilla.com and watch what happens.

Answering a different question

If given an option, we tend to follow the path that requires the least effort. We often answer questions without much scrutiny as to whether the answer is truly appropriate, or we answer an easier question without noticing we have done so. Alternatively, we attempt to answer the question with an answer that seems intuitively to be correct, as it is easier to do so than to stop and think about it.

An example of answering a different question: "A bat and a ball cost $1.10. The bat is one dollar more than the ball. How much is the ball?" If you answered "10 cents" you are incorrect. 10 cents is the instinctive answer to the question, even though 5 cents is the correct answer. This example is taken from Daniel Kahneman's great work *Thinking, Fast and Slow*.

This kind of reasoning occurs at work as much as it does in general conversation and in trick mathematics questions. We see a situation and interpret what we hear, what we see and what is being asked of us in the workplace. I have had the uncomfortable circumstance on at least one occasion where I have been asked to do something by my boss, have gone off and done what I thought he wanted and come back only to be told "What did you do that for? That is not what I asked you to do." The issue was that I did not listen effectively enough, made an assumption as to what was required and went off and did it. I had answered a different question; one that I thought would do the trick. Oops, I got it wrong. Keep an eye on this when you are seeing differences between what someone says they were asked to do and what the task assigner believes they asked to be done.

It is for this reason that when we have conversations, assign tasks or try to understand an incident, we need to listen generously and seek clarification of how a situation really is. Stop and think about what is being asked of us, and what we are asking.

There are a couple of areas related to 'answering a different question' within incidents and incident investigations. The first is with regards to task allocation by the supervisor. I have come across many examples where a worker is carrying out a task that they believe the supervisor wanted them to do, but then a conversation with the relevant supervisor reveals a different story: "I did not tell them to do that. I told them…"

Do not assume automatically that either the supervisor or the worker is lying. It could easily be a case of the worker answering a different question.

The other area where 'answering a different question' plays a part is during post-incident interviews. As I said in Chapter 2, it is quite common for those still in the learning process of interviewing to be poor at listening. They may be too focussed on the questions they are asking, rather than listening in order to understand the answers being given. So the person being interviewed may answer a different question and it is not picked up by the interviewer. A simple trick to help you avoid this is to ask yourself a question each and every time you ask a question at work. Ask yourself, "Did that response actually answer the question I asked?"

> **For your consideration:**
>
> Consider your own experiences. After completing a task set by your superior, have you ever come back to them only to be told that what you did was not asked for?
>
> During your next few meetings, sit back and listen to people 'answering a different question'. It is a lot more common than you may think.

What-You-See-Is-All-There-Is and Plan Continuation

What-You-See-Is-All-There-Is was coined by Daniel Kahneman and is one of those cognitive biases that we all experience. Plan Continuation is another bias and talked about often in relation to NASA and aviation incidents. They both apply to much more than this and were present in many of the serious incidents that I have investigated, if only by knowing what to look for. Biases along with heuristics are those human things that directly impact our decision-making processes. In the case of What-You-See-Is-All-There-Is, we assume, quite subconsciously, that what we see is all that we need to see, particularly when we are mapping out the scenario that could lead to a certain, or expected, outcome.

We create stories about how the world around us operates, often to the detriment of other potential signals that could open up a new story. This drives us to jump to conclusions which are then much harder to change. We are, according to Kahneman in *Thinking, Fast and Slow*, machines made for jumping to conclusions, which we all do all the time, just to survive and make sense of the world we live in and interact with.

Simply being aware of this trap (and trust me, we all fall into it) leads to questions such as "What is really going here that I am ignoring?" or "Is there something that I am missing, or not seeing here?"

More often than not, conditions change or deteriorate gradually and ambiguously, not suddenly and obviously. In a gradual change, there will almost always be cues that suggest the situation is under control and can be continued without increased risk, or the opposite.

But sometimes we are so intent on the job, so focussed and 'into' the task, that we do not see anything else going on around us. NASA talks about the term Plan Continuation, plan continuation bias or plan continuation error to explain this mindset. Once a person has a plan in place, they start to follow that plan and tend not to change or stop the work, even when small signs emerge indicating they should stop and reconsider. This is often seen in aviation collision with terrain incidents where the benefits of hindsight show us that a go-around seemed to be the best choice, but was not chosen in foresight. We often don't see incremental changes that in hindsight are crystal clear. I have seen it described as the unconscious cognitive bias to continue with the original plan in spite of changing conditions. This can also be thought of as a decision to continue with the original plan despite cues that suggested changing the course of action.

Plan Continuation tends to be more prominent towards the final stages of a task. It can have the effect of obscuring those subtle clues which reveal the flaws in the original plan making it no longer valid. It is important during an investigation that hindsight bias is acknowledged and understood to be playing a role. Remember also that the application of the plan continuation bias does not reflect a right or a wrong way to view a developing incident.

For your consideration:

Collect a handful of incident investigation interviews and reports from your business and examine them for evidence of plan continuation bias and see whether it was picked up by the investigation teams.

Shared space as it relates to safe workspaces

'Shared space' is a way of thinking derived from a traffic-management philosophy. It was created in the Netherlands by Hans Monderman and involves the removal of traffic controls such as stop signs, traffic lights, speed limits, pedestrian crossings, barriers and gates, caution and warning signs, painted lines between different traffic users and so on. The idea is to increase the unease of road users and encourage mutual respect and communication – either direct or indirect, including eye contact and visual cues – in order for all road and intersection users to interact safely and effectively.

While shared space has some detractors – and also has some overenthusiastic supporters who claim it to be the best thing since sliced bread – its links and opportunities to safety are significant, although not yet well explored.

Over many years, after many pedestrian and vehicle interactions and accidents, countless traffic controls have crept into our driving and walking lives. But in the concept of shared space, the vast majority of these are removed. The idea is based on voluntary behavioural change of all users, supported by clever space design and implied understanding of how to use the space. In effect, the controls are removed and the people using the system become reliant on each other to remain safe.

Imagine for a moment, if you will, a worksite where the myriad of safety signs (especially those deemed "stupid" or "stating the obvious" by your people) have been removed, and everyone using the area is fully aware of the hazards, the risks and the controls they need to implement before they are free to interact. In this kind of zone, observation skills become very important. It reminds me of James Reason's idea of 'feral vigilance', or the idea of chronic unease that many modern safety science thinkers talk about. The need to be mindful, or aware of what is going on and not to rely on signs and lines painted on the ground. A few words about being mindful and the concept of mindfulness is useful here. Although it seems to be a bit of a flavour of the month at the moment and although the modern usage of the word 'mindfulness' does not feel the same as its Buddhist roots, it is a useful thought process. Weick, Sutcliffe and Obstfeld say in their piece *Organizing for High Reliability: Processes of Collective Mindfulness*, "Mindfulness… is as much about what people do with what they notice as it is about the activity of noticing itself."

Of course, not all workspaces are amenable to the level of control, or lack of it, described within the idea of shared space, but it is absolutely worth exploring as a contributor to an incident. In my experience, over-reliance on or blindly following signs can increase the risk of an incident occurring.

I am not encouraging the wholesale removal of controls – I am merely stating that we should look both before an incident, during our day-to-day work and also after an incident to check if we have overdone the controls. We do not want to dumb down our people by encouraging them to be reliant on signage.

Is allowing people to have some level of discomfort and encouragement to think before they act such a bad thing? And thinking about whether all of this is contained within an environment and system that is tolerant of mistakes being made. We know that failures will occur. Have we created an environment where we can fail safely? Because fail we will.

As usual, a balance needs to be struck. We often hear complaints that the practice of 'safety' means wrapping people up in cotton wool, with a long list of procedures and processes that cause workers to stop thinking for themselves about what could go wrong and what they must do to prevent it going wrong. This is essentially where the thinking behind shared space intersects with the designing or building of safe work. It is also a prompt to help us think about what level of overprotection played a part in an incident or a workplace situation.

Not only should we look out for too many signs in the workplace, but also whether they actually add value or not. I recall one beautifully created sign that had probably cost a small fortune, as it had been placed on all of the rest-room doors on all floors in a very large office I worked in. Its message? It was advising users not to drink the water out of the toilet bowls. This was in a very modern office tower in Perth, the state capital city of Western Australia… this is simply a dumb sign.

For your consideration:

Go for a long and slow walk around your workplace and observe the signage and the messages they may be sending. And then get rid of half of them.

Effective 'core competency training' and 'awareness induction'

Let's do a quick recap on the differences between inductions and core competency training. Inductions are all about raising awareness in the people exposed to the risks of the workplace so that they have cause to stop and think before barging off in a direction they may later regret. To be more specific, imagine an induction workshop in which the presenter shows a picture of an elevated work platform. They then say:

> Here is an elevated platform where you may need to stand when carrying out certain tasks. But before we let you do that, we need to take you through some safety hoops. Even though a 2 metre drop may not seem too significant to you at this moment, in actual fact if you disregarded the safety rules I am about to talk about, you could fall and seriously injure yourself, or at the extreme, you could die.

This is a good induction conversation.

Core competency training is a whole different ball game. It is about making absolutely sure that the person being trained knows what to do in their job. Moreover, they have proven they can do it through effective competency assessments. Classroom-based learning should only make up a small portion of the training, with the remainder more focussed on in-the-field- or on-the-job-based lessons. Such training must always be aligned to the specific work of those involved. In my view it needs to include the topics covered here in this chapter of the book, as well as the essential basics of decision-making, assessing the risks associated with certain jobs, task assignment, problem-solving, communication and handling conflicting requirements. I have seen, and sat through, too many training sessions where a presenter reads the presentation slides out loud and then presents us with a multiple choice 'test'. We review the test as a group and any errors are self-corrected. The tests then all get handed in and everyone participating is deemed competent. What rubbish! If you see any of this in your workplace, get upset about it and do whatever you can to stop it. But, in relation to incident investigations, it is all about asking questions about the training; whether it is competency-based, a simple induction or some combination of the two. Do not make an assumption when you hear or read that a person has been 'trained'. Take the time and check it out.

For your consideration:

Check out your induction. Is it trying to pass itself off as training?

Sit through the induction again. How thorough is the 'competency assessment' at the end? Are the participants simply told the correct answers?

Does your training programme give participants 'true' competency?

When doing an incident investigation, take a small diversion and check out the quality of your induction and training processes, and how they may have contributed to someone's decision-making processes.

Individual actions and assessments

People base all of their actions on their view of the world at that point in time and space. This might seem logical, but it is often overlooked when we are analysing the decision-making process that played a part in an incident. I want to differentiate this section from the one on sense-making I covered earlier. They are related, but worth separating and thinking about slightly differently when exploring what is driving an individual's actions.

When things do not always go to plan, we tend to start looking at people's 'assessments' and people's 'actions'. I believe, as I have mentioned before, that we should be exploring these 'assessments' and 'actions' all the time, not just when we have an unintended outcome. Actions are what people did that failed to produce the expected result, or which produced an unintended outcome or consequence. Assessments are related to how a situation appeared, such as how a person or team viewed a problem prior to a decision or (erroneous) action being taken.

If you are investigating an incident, then understanding the actions of the individual involved is critical – they have a different view of the world than you do, particularly as you only see it after an event has happened (through the eyes of hindsight bias). Erroneous assessments and actions are out there all of the time. It is only rarely that they are seen to cause an unplanned outcome. The vast majority of times erroneous assessments and actions still end up in safe work, or at least end up with an outcome that does not involve an injury or illness. Incidents are very rare. Also remember that people's behaviour is the start of an investigation, not the end of one. It is important to remember at this point that what a person did – the action that led to the incident you are investigating or the work situation you are observing – is not the 'cause' of the incident or situation. It is perfectly acceptable to think about the action that led to the incident as a trigger but not as a cause.

As the work we do and the workplaces we operate in become both more complicated and more complex, the simple notion of 'cause and effect' behind Isaac Newton's third law of motion gets blurred, and the concept of an event having a root cause becomes meaningless.

For your consideration:

When next you are having a conversation with someone about an action they have done, explore how they saw the action and its outcome. Do you see it in the same way?

Systems of work and their interrelationships

To further understand a particular individual's actions, we can explore how the systems interacted with each other and impacted that individual. As we discussed in the section on procedural complexity, it is often the case that within one procedure there is confusion and a lack of clarity and direction. When you get five or ten procedures that must be followed in order to get a job done, this lack of clarity can be amplified exponentially and can become complex.

When an incident occurs, it is often the interaction of the systems that makes the difference, not only one system or process on its own.

Here we are talking about how effectively all the normal systems we would see in a safety management system exist and interact with each other. Some examples of systems that often interact in an incident include systems such as permit to work, contractor management, management of change, legal requirements, risk management, confined space, working at height and traffic management. The question is whether these systems are sound and whether they are interacting with each other in a way that has contributed to the gaps we are exploring between Work-As-Done, Work-As-Normal and Work-As-Intended.

Another set of factors to consider comes from the work of Hollnagel on FRAM. FRAM stands for Functional Resonance Analysis Method and is a stand-alone investigation method. It is very well described in his book of the same name. From our perspective the take-aways from FRAM are related to thinking about the incident as a variability within and between a set of functions that relate to the tasks under investigation. He suggests in his book that "It is more important to understand the nature of system dynamics and the variability of performance, than to model individual, technological or human failures." The FRAM describes the functions that are required for a system to work as it is intended to work. There are six aspects for each of these functions that are examined. These are what are of interest to us here as they are a great way of thinking about work. They are Input, Output, Precondition, Resource, Control and Time. Hollnagel defines them in *FRAM – the Functional Resonance Analysis Method: Modelling Complex Socio-Technical Systems* as follows:

- Input: that which the function processes or transforms or that which starts the function.
- Output: that which is the result of the function, either an entity or a state change.
- Preconditions: conditions that must exist before a function can be carried out.
- Resources: that which the function needs when it is carried out (execution condition) or consumes to produce the Output.
- Control: how the function is monitored or controlled.
- Time: temporal constraints affecting the function (with regard to starting time, finishing time or duration).

As you explore your incident consider how these aspects may have played a part and varied between how they were intended to work and how they actually worked during the incident.

For your consideration:

Have a look at a task being done today by your team. See if you can work out which systems are in play and whether they all align or not.

It is all obvious when you know the outcome (hindsight bias)

In *The Field Guide to Understanding 'Human Error'*, Dekker states: "One of the safest bets you can make as an investigator is that you know more about the incident than the people who were caught up with it – thanks to hindsight." He also says "Hindsight changes how we look at past decision-making. It turns real, convoluted complexity into a simple linear story."

Once a workplace incident has happened and we hear about it, we build this "simple linear story" very quickly in our minds, usually completely at the subconscious level.

It is easy for us to believe this simple linear story after the incident has occurred. But that story did not exist at the time of the incident. We have only created it in hindsight. What existed at the time of the incident is the world-view, the perspective, of those involved at the time. It is worth remembering that even those involved directly in an incident will suffer from the hindsight bias when they are looking back on the incident and are trying to understand it. We need to get firmly into the shoes of the person, or people, involved. We need to explore what perspective they had as the incident unfolded.

Remember that the perspective taken at the time – the view of how the world looks – will greatly affect the decision-making process in the various 'assessments' identified.

For your consideration:

Examine your own thoughts next time you are told about a workplace incident. Examine how much hindsight bias is playing a part in your views and in what you say.

Accountability and authority mismatch

These days there seems to be a significant industry push to hold people to account for their actions, particularly after something has gone wrong. Before jumping on board with this thinking, stop for a moment – and ask yourself a few questions: Did the people you are holding accountable have the authority to make decisions about their work? Did they have the capability and authority to carry out the work the way you believe it should be done? And how were you planning to hold them accountable anyway?

It adds zero value to an investigation to announce that one person was accountable for the actions they undertook, and it was by their decision and choice that the incident occurred. We need to explore in what way they had the authority – explicit or implicit – that supported their decisions, assessments and actions. Real work, on a day-to-day basis is absolutely full of accountability/authority mismatches.

The idea of Work-As-Done and Work-As-Intended ties in very well with the idea of accountability/authority mismatch. We know that the way work is done does not always match the way we intend it to be done and we know that people need to do work that is not always aligned with procedures. If we subscribe to the 'compliance to procedures is absolute' school of work and we suffer an incident we can then hold people accountable for failing to follow a procedure. What about everybody else who are also not following that particular procedure, every single day? What about the people who wrote the procedure that is not able to be followed? We need to impart authority in individuals to make the changes required to complete the work. It is only when there is a match between what we want to hold someone to account for and their requisite authority, that can we hold people accountable.

> **For your consideration:**
>
> Read through some of your procedures and check out where they list people's responsibilities, and explore whether they give people the authority to take on that accountability.
>
> When carrying out a workplace incident investigation, ask the team to consider whether the individuals really had the power to take on the accountability given to them.

Equipment, tools and plant design

One area that often gets forgotten during both simple Outcome Analyses and in more detailed incident investigations is that of the equipment and tools we ask people to use and the design of the workspace we want them to work in. Determining to what level the equipment, tools and plant design were optimal and created a workplace where it was possible to work safely to begin with is an essential component of any workplace incident investigation.

There is more than one way to open a jar whose lid is on too tight. You can tap the lid on a solid table a bit to loosen it up. You can run the lid under hot water to make it expand and thus become loose. You can use a specially designed tool that looks like a giant pair of pliers – there are lots of ways to skin a cat.

It is the same with creating safe work in your business. The job of the leader on a day-to-day basis, or the investigator after an incident, is to explore if the equipment and tools being used were the correct ones for the specific task, if they were used as designed or not. For example, many home owners use a screwdriver to open tins of paint. This works, usually, but it is not the right tool. You can buy little paint tin openers.

It is often difficult to determine whether the tools and equipment are the right ones and this is where the concept of Work-As-Normal comes into the picture again where you can explore what tools and equipment others use. Sometimes you need to expand this conversation to outside your organization. The internet has proven useful in this capacity for me before.

The bottom line here is to use the investigation team to really challenge the status quo around the equipment, tools and even the design of the workplace when trying to understand an incident.

For your consideration:

Go for a walk. Is your workplace designed in such a way that supports the carrying out of safe work? Or does it set people up to fail, to take short cuts, to miss steps in their creation of safe work?

Do the people doing the work know what tools and equipment are available for them to use, or are they making do with whatever is at hand?

Task planning, assignment, acceptance and monitoring

To maximize the likelihood that a task will be undertaken effectively with the desired production and safety outcomes, some effort needs to go into setting it up for success. It needs to be understood and then planned in such a way as to take into consideration what is going on around the task, who is going to carry out the task, what tools and equipment are available, what procedures or other specific instructions need to be in play and what time restrictions may be appropriate.

One of the best documents I have seen to explain to supervisors, planners and managers what is required when a task is undertaken is called the Safe Task Management Standard and covers the areas of task planning, task assignment, task acceptance and task monitoring along with other elements. Even if your organization does not have such a process, the ideas are applicable for all safe work creation.

Explore, as you create your timelines and explanations for gaps and differences between Work-As-Done, Work-As-Normal and Work-As-Intended, what level of effective task assignment was undertaken.

Don Ash, of 100 small things (www.100smallthings.com.au) talks about a great process for task assignment called CPORT. This process describes the elements of an effective task assignment. CPORT stands for Context, Purpose, Output, Resources and Timeframes. Explore whether these elements were in place during the investigation. In other words, did the person doing the job know the big picture stuff around the task? Did they understand why they needed to do the job, what the expected output of the task was, what resources they could use to get the task done and the timing expectation of the supervisor?

Once the job was under way, was there a process such as field leadership in place, that requires leaders to go into the workplace and formally explore how the tasks are being undertaken, whether the risks are being managed and whether Work-As-Done matches Work-As-Intended?

For your consideration:

What process do you currently use to ensure tasks are planned, assigned and accepted to minimize miscommunication and risk?

Leadership

Where does one start with the topic of leadership? It is such a huge field and one that could easily fill a library.

'Leadership' covers not only the words of those giving instructions, but also their expectations, goals, values, key performance indicators, behaviours and conversations as well. The leader plays an enormous part in the creation of safe work and hence in the prevention of incidents. Therefore, leadership also plays an enormous role as you explore explanations for how and why an incident occurred. I am not going to expound on all the aspects of leadership here. They are amply covered elsewhere. I refer you to the works of Goffee and Jones, Simon Sinek, L. David Marquet, Kim and Mauborgne, Bill George, and also Brynjolfsson and McAfee listed in the Bibliography. The key here is for you to consider the aspects of the leadership, and the impact that leadership has had on those involved as perceived by those involved in the incident, and see whether and how they may have played a part.

Below is a list of some of the areas that may be of interest as you explore the impact leadership has had on work and on the incident of interest:

- How the leaders set and communicate expectations.
- The leaders' perspectives and the reality around procedural compliance.
- The leaders' in-the-field behaviour and frequency.
- The leaders' understanding of the relationship between rules, risk awareness, risk intelligence and safety.
- The key performance indicators and their impact on the team and their behaviour.
- The leaders' level of interest in safety and incident investigations.
- Whether the leaders believe/think that safety incidents are caused or created.
- The leaders' views on whether following the rules or doing the right thing is more important.
- The leaders' views on who should be held accountable after a safety event – the operator who did not follow the rules and got it wrong, or the dude who wrote and approved the procedure that was not easy to follow.
- The leaders' views on how you decide when a production or cost initiative impacts safety.
- How the leaders monitor procedural drift over time in the operation.
- The line between what is acceptable and unacceptable behaviour.
- The balance between critiquing errors and celebrating successes.
- If failures are OK if they fail safely (e.g. an object dropped into an exclusion zone).
- Whether the leaders believe people are a problem to solve or a solution to harness.
- Whether leaders investigate incidents to learn or to blame.
- The leaders' belief in the safety system as sufficient to ensure safety.

For your consideration:

What are your leadership models at work and are they conducive to enhancing the quality and purpose of incident investigations?

Convert the bullet points above this box into questions and ask them of your leadership even when you have not just had a workplace incident.

Other cognitive biases and heuristics

A heuristic is, roughly speaking, a rule of thumb which we all use every day to help us make decisions. The use of, or reliance on, a heuristic produces a bias in judgement. They work by reducing complexity. Heuristics are sometimes referred to as mental shortcuts used to help us solve a problem. In and of themselves, they are essential for us to get through the day. As an example, consider the representative heuristic, where we compare the present situation to a representative mental example that then enables us to make a quicker judgement or decision. You need to decide whether to trust someone or not. A sweet, older woman who looks a bit like your granny is likely to come across to you as more trustworthy than a younger, rough-looking man. This is a heuristic at work. It could be correct and aid you or it could be completely wrong. This is where the resultant bias comes in.

Biases are systematic errors and can be viewed as deviations from rational decision-making. In an example that Kahneman uses in *Thinking, Fast and Slow*, when a handsome and confident speaker comes to the stage, the audience will tend to judge his comments more favourably than he deserves. The availability of a diagnostic label for this bias – the halo effect – makes it easier to anticipate, recognize and understand.

There are many ways in which we can describe the explanations for why we do not behave as rational decision-makers as some economic models would have us do. Unfortunately, some people view those involved in workplace incidents as rational decision-makers and that the decisions they made prior to, and during an incident are the reason for, or the cause of, the incident in question. This is a direct result of many of the biases that are discussed in the literature and some of which we will talk about here. Of the hundreds of biases described, I have chosen a dozen that I feel are the most relevant to our needs in understanding workplace incidents. They are worth understanding and thinking about.

Availability bias

The availability bias is a tendency to overestimate the likelihood of an event when the event, or one similar to it, is fresh in your memory. The availability bias also kicks in if the remembered event is unusual or emotionally charged. Over time the impact of the availability bias fades. For example, after a workplace fall from height incident, workers tend to overestimate the likelihood of a fall in their THAs and risk assessments. This can result in the fall risk taking precedence over other, more relevant risks that need to be controlled in a given circumstance. Some control may be missed and we end up with a workplace incident that did not have anything to do with working at height. An example from the health arena is where a recent experience with a disease by a physician may inflate the likelihood of a misdiagnosis in a current case.

Completeness bias

In some ways, the completeness bias is related to Daniel Kahneman's What-You-See-Is-All-There-Is (from *Thinking, Fast and Slow*), where decisions are made without consideration of all the data needed. In the case of the completeness bias, the information presented, either in a written or a verbal form, seems to be definitive and all aspects seem to have been well covered and so a decision is made. It is often only after the fact, using the hindsight bias, that we see things that were missed.

Two examples related to workplace incidents and their investigations come to mind. The first is related to the risk assessment created prior to an incident in order to identify the hazards and required controls. When looking at risk assessments either before an incident or after an incident during an investigation, they are often found wanting in their hazard identification details. This is often due to the completeness bias, where those creating the risk assessment got to the point of saying "we have finished" too early in the process.

The other example relates to the reviewing of gathered data during a detailed incident investigation. On many occasions, a well-meaning safety or operational/managerial person gathers a pile of paperwork and information that they think the investigation team will need and then presents the information to the team at the start of the data-gathering phase of the investigation. I do not allow the investigation team to look over any of this collected information until they have completed the PEEPO step of the investigation (see Chapter 3) and have worked out what information they want to collect for themselves. If they use the information already collected for them, the completeness bias kicks in and they feel they have enough information to get going with. This usually results in a biased investigation outcome that misses important information. It is only through the investigation team thinking for themselves about what information and data they need in order for them to understand the incident that helps reduce the completeness bias during this part of the investigation.

Confirmation bias

The confirmation bias is a very human way of thinking, as are many of the cognitive biases we are covering here. It occurs when people selectively focus on data and evidence that support their belief of a situation at the time, at the expense of data and evidence that does not support their belief or view.

Prior to an incident, a work team may selectively incorporate ideas and risks that support the carrying out of the task in a certain way and ignore ideas and risks that could scupper the plan during a risk assessment. This is a classic example of the confirmation bias at work. Another is when a medical practitioner looks for confirming evidence to support a diagnosis rather than looking for evidence that does not support the diagnosis. This is not an intentional omission, just one driven from the existence of the confirmation bias.

Taking a step back from the activity and reconsidering the facts can help minimize the confirmation bias, as can carrying out a pre-mortem on what could go right and what could go wrong.

Control bias (illusion of control)

We tend to overestimate our level of influence over events. From *Risk Intelligence: How to Live with Uncertainty*, Evans says "Psychologists have long known that the illusion of control is a key factor in risk perception; it is probably one of the main reasons why people feel safer driving than when flying, even though driving is more dangerous." The illusion of control bias also plays a major role in safety generally and in incident analysis specifically.

We write procedures and feel that we have control over the behaviours of those using the procedure as a result. We carry out workplace incident investigations and come up with 'causes' and corrective actions, as though these are real and will make a difference; that we have control, completely understand what went on and what we need to do to 'fix it'. This is the control bias at work.

I feel that the illusion of control is one of the drivers of managers feeling the need to create corrective actions for all workplace incidents, no matter what the incident was or what lay behind it. They feel that the creation of the actions gives them control over a situation that they may not want to admit they do not have complete control over.

At the level of the events that lead to a workplace incident, the illusion of control impacts how those doing the work decide what hazards exist and how they plan to control them. It also impacts their view of the likelihood of things going right, and what impact their work may have on others around them. Watch out for this when you are trying to understand incidents in your workplace.

Escalation bias

This bias is the driver of Plan Continuation, which is sometimes declared as a bias in its own right. (We have talked about Plan Continuation in another section in this chapter.) If you walked into the middle of a task as it was unfolding, would you be able to see what escalation was going on? We are often blind to the subtle cues and changes that go on in our environment as we carry out our work. As we progress through the tasks, things change but we do not register them as being sufficiently important to change our plans. It is very hard to see escalation bias at the time. It is easy to see after something has not worked out the way we thought it was going to (with hindsight bias kicking in).

Framing effect

Depending on whether data are presented to us as positive data or as negative data, we tend to make different decisions. People, including those directly involved in any workplace situation or incident you may be investigating, will tend to prefer the sure thing over the gamble (they are risk-averse) when the outcome seems good and they tend to reject the sure thing and accept the gamble (they are risk-seeking) when the outcome is stated, or framed, as negative. This has an impact on how a task is set up prior to, or during an incident and reinforces the idea of focussing on those things that make things go right rather than focussing on trying to minimize what might go wrong.

The framing effect can manifest during an incident as the THA is being prepared. Depending on how the consequences are framed will impact the likelihood of that step being undertaken with those consequences. A certain result framed as a positive is much easier to decide upon than a certain result framed as a negative. The reverse is true for risky decisions.

Fundamental Attribution Effect

Todd Conklin, in *Pre-Accident Investigations: An Introduction to Organizational Safety*, tells a great story that sums up the Fundamental Attribution Effect extremely well:

> "A worker is walking across the office parking lot to go in to his office. During this walk, the worker steps on a rock and sprains his ankle. The injury is bad enough that the worker has to go to the clinic and have his leg treated. The worker ends up with a series of x-rays, a cast on his foot, and a day or two off from work.

This is an example of an error; however, this error will be attributed to the worker's judgement and walking ability. At some point, some manager will comment that if this worker had "watched where he was going" this event would not have happened. If this worker had cared more, the worker would have been more attentive. If the worker had been more attentive, the worker would have stepped over the rock, and completely avoided this injury. The injury is clearly the worker's fault. The organization is attributing the error to the worker's judgement and behavioural choices. In a way, what the organization will do is assume that a bad outcome must happen to a bad person. You will hear some manager say something like this, "if only... the worker would have paid more attention". Read on and see how remarkably unfair that way of thinking is to your workforce.

> The next day, the manager of the "twisted ankle worker" who was injured the day before was walking across the same parking lot.
>
> The manager had a lot on her mind. She had a reportable injury. She had a worker who had had to go to the hospital and get medical attention. She had an employee that had got hurt under her watchful eye. While this manager was thinking of all these things she stepped on a rock, the very same rock, in the parking lot, and twisted her ankle. She was in pain and could barely walk... but she didn't report the injury. Instead, this manager found out whose job it was in her organization to sweep the parking lots and sidewalks. The manager immediately called the roads and grounds crew supervisor, and had his crew sweep the parking lot. Because this manager was so busy thinking about the event that had happened to her worker, she was concentrating on her safety problem and not on where she was walking.

What is intriguing about this concept is the idea that when the worker walked incorrectly it was the worker's fault. When the manager walked badly, her response was to not only fix the problem, but also to move the fault from her as the manager to the person whose job it was to keep rocks off the parking lot."

This is the fundamental attribution error in action. It is extremely common for people after a workplace incident to attribute people's behaviour to their core character rather than to their situation. A way to help overcome this as you hear about an incident is to ask "What is responsible for this incident?" rather than "Who is responsible for this incident?" Try to remember that what looks like a people problem is often a situation problem.

Gambler's Fallacy

"I've done this task a thousand times and nothing has ever happened before. I don't understand why it went so wrong this time" is a common response to an incident. "We have gone 300 days without a recordable injury. Surely we can easily get to a year injury free. Then we can really celebrate." Both of these statements are classic examples of the Gambler's Fallacy. The Gambler's Fallacy is described as the tendency to think that the future likelihood of an outcome is impacted by past events, when in reality it is not. During an investigation, ask those involved about how they assessed the risk of some task going right or going wrong. If they look back in time and say that it has always gone well when we did it that way, this should pique your interest in exploring whether the Gambler's Fallacy is playing a part in the decision-making process.

One solution to the Gambler's Fallacy is to stop and look at a situation from different angles, rather than just through the lens of the past and how that has worked out for you.

Neglect of Probability

The Neglect of Probability bias is all about being binary; 0 or 1, black or white, something will or something will not happen, even though the actual outcome is uncertain. Watch out for the Neglect of Probability bias when reviewing THAs and people are explaining to you the logic they used in its creation. Listen for "That could never happen" as compared to "That outcome is unlikely but let's look at it anyway." The first is full of the Neglect of Probability and the latter understands that there is uncertainty in most of what we do.

Outcome bias

Outcome bias refers to the influence of the outcome of an event or situation upon an evaluation of the quality of a decision. It is related to the hindsight bias but should not be confused with it as they are different. The outcome bias shows up as "Bad outcomes must come from bad decisions." Practically this means that we tend to judge a decision by the outcome rather than on the quality of the decision at the time it was made. We have all seen good processes lead to bad outcomes and bad processes lead to good outcomes. This is in fact a major driver for a difference between Work-As-Done and Work-As-Intended. Because workplace incidents are rare, we assume as a result of the outcome bias that good decisions and processes have led to 999 out of 1,000 activities. This is an erroneous use of cause and effect.

As an incident investigation team, it is very important that you try to avoid both the hindsight bias and the outcome bias during the investigations. This can be achieved by trying to remove, to the extent that you can, knowledge of the actual outcome during any assessment of decision-making quality. I heard recently of a very senior manager announce to a meeting of other managers at a large organization that he had recently undertaken a review of the last five or six very serious workplace incidents and all of them had been the result of poor choices and decisions made by those who were injured. This is a classic example of the outcome bias at work. In many cases, the outcome bias causes employees and leaders involved in a workplace incident to be blamed for a negative outcome even when they had good intentions and had gone through a sound decision-making process both before and during the development of the incident.

Francesca Gino, from the Harvard Business School, in an article entitled "What We Miss When We Judge a Decision by the Outcome", describes a study which sums up the outcome bias well. In the scenario she describes an evaluation of the decision quality between two conditions. In the test, the two drugs chosen were considered equally effective during clinical trials with one being cheaper than the other:

- A physician prescribed the cheaper drug to save the patient money. Despite the good intentions, the patient suffered from adverse side effects and spent the night in hospital.
- A physician prescribed the more expensive drug in order to generate more revenue for the medical clinic in which he had an interest. Although the physician had selfish intentions, the patient made a full recovery without side effects or hospitalization.

The participants, when looking at both of these situations, rated the selfish physician higher than the one with good intentions. This is a classic case of the outcome bias.

Peltzman Effect (risk compensation)

Two Formula 1 racing cars are sitting on the grid at the Monza F1 circuit preparing to race each other around the 5.8 km track. The one on the inside is a fully kitted-out car with all the safety gear including his six-point seat belt, HANS device (which protects the head and neck of the driver in an accident), fire-suppression system, etc. and the driver is wearing all of the fire-retardant clothing racing suit, helmet and gloves. The car on the outside of the track has the fire-suppression system deactivated, no

HANS device, no seat belts and the driver is wearing a pair of shorts and a tee shirt. Otherwise, the cars are identical F1 cars. The race starts. Who do you think is likely to push the envelope of the cars in terms of grip and win the one-lap race around Monza? You guessed it. The car with all the safety equipment in place and effective. This is what the Peltzman Effect is all about.

The Peltzman Effect is seen when people adjust their behaviour in a way that counteracts the intent of the safety devices installed. It is the driver of "shared space" that we have already talked about. Some things to think about as you carry out an investigation after a workplace incident or as you think about how work is normally done include asking whether you have wrapped up your workers in cotton wool by the mandating of procedures, personal protective equipment, rules, standards and other systems used to control their behaviour to the extent that they think they are safe because they have so many layers of defence that nothing can go wrong. If your people believe that they are safe if they follow all the rules, then this is a dangerous place to be in and one that you need to be inquisitive about as you carry out your incident investigation.

Planning fallacy

This manifests during maintenance shutdown activities across many industries in addition to examples of estimating patient load and nursing staffing levels in healthcare facilities. The planning fallacy is the propensity of people to underestimate the amount of time it will take to complete a task or a series of tasks. It has a direct bearing on safety as it is capable of inducing significant 'production pressure' in the workplace. Of course, we can look at publicly funded projects just about anywhere to see examples of the planning fallacy but it is the impact it can have on safety and workplace incidents that is of interest to us here. As you undertake an incident investigation, have a close look at the planning stages and processes related to the tasks being undertaken at the time of the incident. Questions to ask include: Was the work achievable in the time frame allocated? And were any emergent work or upsets on the tasks such as high-load patients on a ward were taken into consideration or allowed for?

The Efficiency–Thoroughness Trade-Off

We talked briefly about ETTO earlier in this book in relation to the level of investigation we should use for a given workplace incident. We want to focus here more on the ETTO principle as it relates to the work being undertaken at the time of the incident.

In virtually all we do, whether at work or at home, we make a choice that tries to strike a balance between being efficient and being thorough. According to Hollnagel, in *The ETTO Principle – Efficiency–Thoroughness Trade-Off: Why Things that Go Right Sometimes Go Wrong*, "Efficiency means that the level of investment or amount of resources used or needed to achieve a stated goal objective are kept as low as possible." The balance of this is 'thoroughness'. "Thoroughness means that an activity is carried out only if the individual or organization is confident that the necessary and sufficient conditions for it exist so that the activity will achieve its objective and not create any unwanted side-effects." So, it becomes very clear that we cannot be efficient and thorough at the same time; there needs to be a balance, a compromise.

The fact that workplace incidents occur only rarely can mean that Work-As-Normal through the influence of procedural drift can lead the balance to shift over time towards the 'efficiency' side of the balance. Thinking back to the NASA Columbia Space Shuttle foam-shedding catastrophe, here we see the foam-shedding incidents becoming an 'acceptable risk' and not a flight safety issue. This is being efficient in helping turn around the shuttle for the next launch. This happened over and over again through the life of the spacecraft and can be compared to being 'thorough' from the start, where NASA may have investigated and understood the issue before it ended in disaster.

In all levels of workplace incident investigations, it is worth trying to understand the balance between efficiency and thoroughness and what the ETTO balance actually was. The ETTO balance can be at an individual level and also at an organizational level. Work procedures, standards, work instructions and other systems can all show examples of the ETTO principle at work. Explore them as you investigate the incident.

Note

1 Much of this is taken from "Resilience Engineering: New Directions for Measuring and Maintaining Safety in Complex Systems, Final Report December 2008" by Sidney Dekker, Erik Hollnagel, David Woods and Richard Cook and also Hollnagel's *Resilience Engineering in Practice: A Guidebook*.

5   Conclusion

Incident investigations are about the future, not the past. Incident investigations are all about learning. It is paramount to have a focus on how we normally work, how we think we work and how we worked on the day of the incident. Contrary to the historical view, it is actually destructive to put too much focus on who did what that was wrong, or in contravention of a procedure. Taking this a step further, we realize that the idea of Work-As-Done and Work-As-Intended is also embedded in how we set critical controls for our fatal risks.

A good summary of the whole mindset approach to safety and to incident investigations in particular lies with a story about a milking stool: a milking stool has three legs. If you remove one it will fall over. Safety has three legs. If you remove one it will fall over.

Milking stools, or any other three-legged stools for that matter, are very stable when all the legs are in place and working and are held together solidly by the seat part of the stool. It falls over very quickly if any component is defective or missing. They are pretty stable though, even when the ground is uneven. They can handle a bit of uncertainty and even when the legs are a little bit different in length are still able to stand and be effective.

So it is with safety. The three legs that need to be in place to create safe work are: risk intelligence, authentic field leadership and incident investigations. Holding this all together are the conversations we have. Conversations are in many ways the seat of the stool. Without it, we do not even have a stool and it all falls over.

Let's have a look at each in turn.

Risk intelligence is not the same as risk management, risk assessment, risk aversion or risk control. According to Dylan Evans in his book by the same name, risk intelligence is the ability to estimate probabilities and likelihoods accurately. Having our people capable of simply taking a look at what they are about to do and thinking about what could go right as well as what could go wrong, the likelihood of either happening and then deciding what they are going to actually do to make sure it all goes well is what it is all about. Dr Robert Long also talks about the word 'risk' as being interchangeable with the word 'learning' in his thought-provoking book *Real Risk*. I agree. We do not want to be risk-averse in the workplace. That dumbs down risk intelligence. We want people to explore new ways of doing things, of undertaking micro-experiments in their work, of thinking about what controls they choose, not being overly reliant on following procedures like brain-dead lemmings, of learning from the work they do on a daily basis and generally being risk intelligent. In reality, we are setting up Work-As-Intended through changes in THA, changes to procedures and work instructions and through 'management of change' in all these areas. It is important to remember here that we need to strike a balance between the recognition that some controls are 'must haves' and an understanding that these 'must haves' are often not enough on their own. We need to implement the 'must haves' in the context of the task and what else is going on. These non-negotiable 'must haves' are often included in the system under categories like material risk, fatal risk or sometimes critical risk. Risk intelligence is about giving license to be creative and improve Work-As-Normal whilst understanding what must be in place.

The second leg of our safety stool is what I will label authentic field leadership. These are the activities (conversations mainly) that leaders undertake in the field on a day-to-day basis with people doing tasks. The intent is to try to understand the gaps between the way work was done on the day (Work-As-Done), how others normally do the work (Work-As-Normal) and how our processes and procedures intend it to be done (Work-As-Intended); and then we work to close the gaps we have identified. In many ways it is a form of verification as to how work is being done. The most powerful piece of advice I can offer here is for the leader to be authentic in their interactions. In the words of Rob Goffee and Gareth Jones in *Why Should Anyone Be Led by You?*, "Be yourself – more – with skill." Showing who you are as a person, as a leader, showing you really care and are absolutely interested in what the team are doing, how they view the world in front of them and exploring with them, their decision-making processes will get you a very long way in authentic leadership in the field and really support and be helpful to your team.

The third leg is incident investigations which are, of course, the main subject of this book. Here we want to explore what is responsible for an outcome not being quite what we expected it to be (someone had got hurt, perhaps). In exactly the same way as we did for authentic field leadership, here we are trying to understand the gaps between the way work was done on the day of the event (Work-As-Done), how others normally do the work (Work-As-Normal) and how our processes and procedures intended it to be done (Work-As-Intended); and then we work to close the gaps we have identified. I have said this often, and will do so again here: "the conversations we have before an incident should be the same as the conversations we have after an incident".

So, how best to summarize the three legs? We want our people to have the competencies, capabilities and capacities to create safety through risk intelligence, our leaders keeping an eye on things through conversations in the field and sound investigation practices when things do go wrong. The secret is how we choose to help our people get really good at conversations.

Keeping an eye on all of that is a must. But what else can we do? What other actions can we take? What behaviours can we exhibit to ensure it all comes together and the conversations we have within any of the three legs looks, sounds and feels the same?

My recommendation to you is to maintain focus and ensure you are very interested in how work is actually being done – not just how we intend the work to be done as set out in our procedures. This is as important before an incident as it is after an incident during an investigation.

That said, we should make sure our procedures, standard operating procedures, work instructions and so on are setting our people up for success. Challenge each process as you explore an incident: Are they able to be followed? Are they simple? Do they make it easy to do things correctly and harder to do them incorrectly? Do they allow for the risk intelligence of the individuals? Do they align with each other? Do they contain elements of resilience? Do they explain the controls that must be implemented, and when? Are they written in the way those who have to use them want them to be written? Are the critical controls from our fatal risks being verified by those who use them? We can use the same language as we build our fatal risk controls as we talk to people in the field, and as we investigate unintended outcomes.

And all of this will help us as we explore the gaps between Work-As-Done, Work-As-Normal and Work-As-Intended, and then seek to close them.

A quick word or two on the processes themselves to wrap up. The process of Outcome Analysis is designed for simple incidents and thus should be kept very simple. The secret is to make sure the people you expect to carry out the process know the process – and not only should they know the context and intent behind the process, they should also be happy to use it to develop simple actions that will help create a safe future.

It is designed for the front-line supervisor level and so needs strong support by the more senior leaders in the business. A culture of openness and caring after an incident is very important here, as this (or its absence) will dramatically impact the quality and nature of the incident investigation's reports.

And remember that the Outcome Analysis process is powerful because it can be used to investigate positive outcomes just as effectively as it can be used to investigate negative outcomes such as safety, health, environmental, financial, process or mechanical failure incidents. You can wield it to explore how you normally do work, to identify where gaps exist between Work-As-Done, Work-As-Normal and Work-As-Intended on a day-to-day basis. You can also apply the science behind it, especially those concepts discussed in Chapter 4 and Appendix A, as a basis for conversations with your people, your leaders and industry groups at any time.

As for more detailed incident investigations, the science behind the process is the same as for Outcome Analyses. The intent is also the same. It is only the depth that varies. The conversations you have to collect information, the timelines, the make-up of the team and the report are all more formal. Other than that, it is the same process.

By far the most important concept that I want to leave you with is mindset. By this, I mean our views, perspectives and the approach in our mind as we hear about workplace incidents and then undertake investigations into them. It really gets back to Simon Sinek's thoughts on starting with Why. Sinek views as critical the need to clearly understand why we do things. Once you understand your 'why', then the application of and the carrying out of the 'what' just happens. This applies to incident investigations just as well as to pretty much anything else. If we spend time thinking about the why of investigating unintended outcomes, whether they are positive or negative outcomes, and we really understand in our minds why approaching an investigation with an intent to understand what is responsible for the outcome rather than who is responsible, then the rest will be simple and will fall into place. Once we know our investigation why, our demeanour will change. Our body language will change. We will come across as caring, eager to understand, empathetic and generally open and honest in our incident investigation style. This is true regardless of the depth or complexity of the incident investigation.

Another point worth taking home is the idea that these methods of incident investigation, whilst based on the latest science and thinking in safety and decision-making, are just models, ideas, approaches. Just like any model, once you understand it in detail; once you get the science and the thoughts that go into it; once you understand your why; only then will you be able to apply it from a position of strength. You will know which bits to pay attention to, which bits to gloss over or ignore completely, and which bits to modify to suit your purposes and your incident specifically. You will have a different approach investigating a medication-related incident in the healthcare arena than you would have whilst investigating a process plant upset in a pigment manufacturing plant, yet the underlying method and thinking is the same. Do not treat this book as a procedure, but rather as a guide, a thought and conversation provoker.

The most important ideas that I believe you need to internalize are resilience along with the concepts of Work-As-Done, Work-As-Normal, Work-As-Intended and procedural drift. I really recommend you get your head around these ideas. Appendix A will also help here, as will a thorough reading of Dekker, Hollnagel and Snook. Of course, I thoroughly recommend all the other books in the Bibliography as well. I hope you enjoyed my book and got something out of it.

Appendix A
Interviewing: having meaningful conversations

The idea of this appendix is to offer you a selection of questions that you may find useful as a guide when you are having conversations with people after an incident, or even before an incident when you are exploring how work is being done and how work is normally done. They are framed as a mixture of open, closed and direct questions and should be used as a guide to conversations, not as a set of questions to fire at someone. The questions are primarily intended to be used during the interview process associated with data-gathering. But I have also found them useful when discussing details with the investigation team, as they help the investigation team think differently about aspects of the incident. The questions are intended to be used in a non-directive way. The way I use these questions during an investigation, whether I am facilitating a fatality or heading up/helping people do some interviews, is that I flip through them before the investigation/interview starts. I do not try to learn them, but find that simply scanning through them sets them up in my mind so that when I am having the conversation the questions are not far beneath the surface of my mind and so float up and become simply a part of the conversations I am having. As discussed in the main body of the book, an interview related to an incident is a conversation and not a list of questions to be answered, which is why I do not support the idea of using this appendix to formulate exactly what questions you will ask. The other benefit of the list is that by reading through the questions, you will get a deeper understanding of the topic and its intent. Put another way, as the interviewer, use the following as a pre-interview guide for yourself. Use your own words and make sure the choice of language is suitable for the interviewee. Above all, remember that this is a conversation.

Align your mind with the interview process and become familiar with what sort of questions may work best during the interview conversations.

Note: there is some duplication of questions as some fit quite well into different categories. In addition, for ease of use, the questions are grouped by topic and then by the PEEPO categories of People, Environment, Equipment, Procedures and Organization.

Communication

People

- Did someone communicate at the right time (not too early or too late)?
- Did the individuals accurately follow a communications procedure?
- Was information communicated accurately?
- Did the person giving instructions verify understanding?
- Did the person receiving instructions ask for clarification?
- Was all relevant information included in the shift change handover?
- Did the person receiving the information pass it on to the key individuals that needed it?
- Were communications clear?
- Were key individuals present during the communication process (to receive/relay information)?
- Did a person correctly use the required communication hardware (e.g. radio, public address system)?
- Was an alarm or display misunderstood?
- How does the leader set and communicate expectations?
- What is the balance between the use of verbal and non-verbal forms of communication?
- How are messages transferred across to those who need them?
- Were messages cascaded accurately?
- What does the leader do and say in the field?
- What is the balance between tell and listen when the leader communicates?
- How does the leader monitor procedural drift over time?
- How are assessments of communication adequacy and effectiveness undertaken?

Environment

- Were communications obscured by noise or other environmental factors?
- Could communications not be sent because the system was busy/overloaded (e.g. radio traffic)?

- Was an alarm or display not heard or seen when it should have been?
- Was the work area so noisy that critical alarms or alerts were difficult to hear?

Equipment

- Was appropriate communication equipment available (e.g. telephones, radios)?
- Was communication equipment fit for purpose?
- Was communication equipment in working order?
- Does the communication equipment permit faults (e.g. users may use the wrong radio channel without noticing)?
- Were there any recent modifications to the plant that rendered the detection/alert system inoperative, ineffective, or that were missed by the alarm system entirely?
- Were instructions or warnings in a different language/non-standard language?

Procedures

- Had the team read all of the procedures that they are supposed to follow for this task?
- What are the formal and informal communications systems at work?
- Are there procedures to ensure timely and effective communications?
- Are the communications-related procedures easy to follow correctly or easier to not follow correctly?

Organization

- Is there a shift change handover process?
- Are supervisors made aware of employee capabilities or not made aware in a timely fashion? (What human resources process worked or failed around communications?)

Leadership

People

- How do the leaders set and communicate expectations?
- What are the leaders' perspectives and the reality around procedural compliance?

- What do the leaders do when they are in the field? What is their behaviour and how often do they go into the field?
- What is the leaders' understanding of the relationship between rules, risk awareness, risk intelligence and safety?
- Do the organization's key performance indicators have an impact on the team and behaviour?
- What is the leaders' level of interest in safety and incident investigations?
- Do the leaders believe/think that safety incidents are caused or created?
- What are the leaders' views on which is more important: following the rules or doing the right thing?
- What are the leaders' views on who should be held accountable after a safety event – the operator who did not follow the rules and got it wrong, or the dude who wrote and approved the procedure?
- How do the leaders monitor procedural drift over time?
- Who draws the line between what is acceptable and unacceptable behaviour?
- Does the leadership believe that failures are OK if the failure ends safely (e.g. an object dropped into an exclusion zone)?
- Do the leaders believe people are a problem to be solved or a solution to harness?
- Why do leaders think they investigate events?
- Do we investigate incidents to learn or to blame?
- Do the leaders believe that the safety system is sufficient to ensure safety?
- What do senior leaders talk with you about when they visit with you in the workplace?
- Are inspections by leaders conducted by checklists subject to "tick and flick" behaviour?
- Was a supervisor able to verify a worker's competency?
- Did the supervisor choose people who were capable of performing the task?
- Were a supervisor's directions or decisions so forceful that everyone complied without question?
- Did a supervisor correct work that was being carried out incorrectly?
- Has a planned task observation been done recently?
- How does the supervisor ensure that procedures were being followed?
- Was the supervisor too focussed on another issue to provide adequate oversight?
- Does the supervisor review and endorse hazard/risk assessments?
- Was a pre-job briefing done at the work site?
- Was the person required to learn on the job but no mentoring or coaching was given?

- What do the leaders think 'safety' is?
- What is the leaders' understanding of the concept of authentic leadership?
- What is the leaders' understanding of the concept of mindful leadership?
- What are the leaders' views on how to decide when a production or cost initiative impacts safety?
- What do the senior managers do to develop their supervisors, superintendents and managers?

Environment

- What were the noise levels (and other distractions) when in-the-field leadership communications were being done?

Equipment

- Has the field leadership process detected any equipment-related issues?
- Have any field leadership process identified equipment-related issues been addressed?

Procedures

- Was a shift change handover process used?
- Is there a formal procedure or system that covers the leaders' roles during shift change handover process? And was it used?
- What are the leaders' views and beliefs associated with procedural compliance?
- How is procedural compliance monitored?

Organization

- Was the supervision span of control sufficient?
- Is there a tolerance for shortcuts?
- Is there a culture of getting things done or a drive for quality and/or adherence to procedure?
- Is there a department or team microculture of exceeding tolerances by "just a little"?
- Is there a process in place to review the performance against leadership styles or expectations?

Resilience and resilience engineering

People

- In the preparation of a Take Five or THA, how much thought did those involved put into what could go wrong?
- In the preparation of a Take Five or THA, how much thought did those involved put into what could go right?
- Which specific parts of a task needed extra vigilance?
- How did those involved prepare their response to expected disruptions?
- What would/did those involved do if something unexpected happens? For example, an interruption, a new and urgent task, an unexpected change of conditions, a resource that is missing.
- Before the team started the task, or during the task, what process did they follow that could have helped them look for and think about any potential disturbances, surprises or changes?
- How did those involved monitor what was going on within the task or around them at the time?
- Did those involved check that there were no disturbances present that might interact with the completion of the task?
- How did the team keep an eye on things that could have become a threat in the near future?
- Did they observe anything that made them think something might not go as planned?
- What was learned since the last time the task was carried out?
- Were there any previous incidents or near misses involving this task or similar tasks?
- Did the THA or procedure encourage people to consider which bits of a task they really needed to pay attention to?
- Did the THA or procedure encourage anyone to plan what the work team 'could' do if something started to go wrong?
- Was the information provided by alarms or displays sufficient?
- Was dismissing or ignoring a display alarm common practice within the department or operation?

Equipment

- Did an alarm fail to go off that should have?

Procedures

- What level of unpredictability arose during the task and how was it managed?

- What do those involved normally do when they are confronted with a situation in which they need to adapt the way they do the task?

Organization

- Does the operation or organization talk about, or have systems for, formal consideration of resilience in their management system?

Risk intelligence, identification and management

People

- Did all of the individuals in the team understand the risks they had described in their THA/Take Five/"Stop and Think"?
- Was the THA done as a group, by an individual, or by the supervisor?
- How realistic are the hazards and hazard controls in the THA?
- In the preparation of the Take Five, how much thought was put into what could go wrong?
- What is the understanding of the risks associated with the job and the required hazard controls?
- Did the team assess the risks for this particular job, and how did they do that?
- What training and guidance, coaching, etc. have occurred with respect to risk intelligence, identification and management?
- What did the team expect to go well?
- What did the team expect to not go well?
- What hazards did the team expect to find?
- What part of the task did the team expect surprises to pop up in?
- Was sufficient risk/hazard identification and assessment conducted prior to the task being undertaken?
- Did an individual or team fail to recognize a hazard because of a lack of experience?

Environment

- What do the team normally do if something unexpected happens in the local environment in which the work is being done?
- Before the team normally starts a task, or during a task, what process do they follow that would, or could help them look for and think about any potential disturbances, surprises or changes in the area that could happen that might impact their work?

- How did those involved monitor what was going on within the task or around them?
- Did the team check that there were no disturbances arising that could have interacted with the completion of the task?

Equipment

- Was correct personal protective equipment for the task available?
- Was wrong or insufficient personal protective equipment identified as mandatory for the task?
- Were protective equipment or devices in place and in working order?
- Was a key defence or barrier missed during a management of change process?

Procedures

- Looking at the THA or work instruction, or procedure, do those involved think it is written in a way that makes it easy to do correctly, or hard to do correctly?
- Is the procedure current in terms of document review?
- Should there have been a procedure for the task but there wasn't?
- Did the bow tie cover the controls that failed in this event?
- Does the procedure form a part of a critical control for a material (or fatal) risk?
- Is the work permit intended to convey information on hazards or risks, but didn't?

Organization

- Did the management of change process alert the person of the presence of a hazard?
- What is the leaders' understanding of the relationship between rules, risk awareness, risk intelligence and safety?
- How does the leader know that all critical controls are in place and effective today, when the tasks are being done?

Systems of work and their interrelationships

People

- What set (or mix) of procedures and systems were in place that were 'supposed' to be followed (e.g. working at height, permit to work, confined space)?

- What differences exist between the systems and procedures that were supposed to be used? (Do all the requirements in the procedures align with each other?)
- Was the change management process properly applied?
- Did the employee have the appropriate licences, certifications or verification of competence?
- Were the people involved trained in the procedure as it currently stands?
- Were those involved deemed competent in the existing procedure?
- Did any key performance indicators have an impact on the team or their behaviour?

Environment

- Was the task affected by simultaneous operations?
- What initiatives are in play right now that might have a disruptive influence on the workplace or on the mindset of those involved?

Equipment

- Did other activities in the area have any impact on the task?
- What do those involved normally do when they are confronted with a situation in which they need to adapt the way they do the task?
- Was a key defence or barrier missed during a management of change process?

Procedures

- Looking at the THA, work instruction or procedure, does the team think it is written in a way that makes it easy to do correctly, or hard to do correctly?
- How consistently is the management of change procedure used?
- Was the work so critical that someone should be supervising work accuracy every time the task is performed, but wasn't?
- Are instructions for performing compliance checks or verifications clear or vague?
- Were the suite of procedures and required documents readily available?
- Are there multiple versions of the procedure available for use?
- Was the procedure able to be followed precisely?
- Were those involved in the task involved in the writing or review of any required procedures or work instructions?

Task complexity, procedural complexity and adequacy and situational complexity

People

- What procedures are in place that leaders expect to be followed?
- How many procedures, standards or work instructions are usually needed to complete the task?
- What is the team's understanding of the procedure?
- Have those involved read the procedure? If so, when?
- What stage of the procedure was the team up to when the incident happened?
- What do the team think about the procedure?
- Is the procedure easy to read and understand?
- Is the procedure easy to follow?
- Looking at the THA, work instruction or procedure, do you think it is written in a way that makes it easy to do correctly, or hard to do correctly?
- What is the level of complexity in the procedure?
- What is the level of complexity in the task?
- How often are the crews included in the review of procedures they are expected to follow?
- Had the team read all of the procedures that they are supposed to follow for this task?
- What level of unpredictability arises during the task and how was it managed?
- Did the person have to leave the alarm unmonitored to complete other job requirements or during breaks?
- Were those involved so overwhelmed by excessive information that important information wasn't detected amongst the 'noise'?
- Did the team miss any key alerts or warnings that indicate they were deviating from a procedure?

Environment

- Were environmental conditions so extreme that housekeeping routines could not keep up/took inordinate amounts of time?

Procedures

- What procedures are in place that were expected to be followed?

- How many procedures, standards or work instructions are usually needed to complete the task?
- Was the procedure overly complicated?

Organization

- Did the document management process fail? If so, in what way?

Task planning, assignment, acceptance and monitoring, including accountability/authority mismatch

People

- What did the team see or notice that was going on around them at the time?
- Was the perspective/view of the situation the same for all team members?
- Did the team seek any guidance as to which way to do the task?
- How confident was the team that what they did was going to work?
- What do those involved normally do if information is missing, or if they cannot get hold of certain people?
- How did the supervisor of this task plan it?
- How did the supervisor of this task assign it to the work team (from the perspectives of the supervisor and the work team)?
- How does the supervisor normally assign tasks?
- What process or thought patterns does the team go through when they have been assigned a task? In other words, what do they do to accept a task from the supervisor?
- How often does the supervisor check in on tasks during the shift?
- Did the supervisor or person in charge provide any preparation (work order, instructions, procedures, etc.) for the work to be performed?
- Was too much work scheduled for the available time?
- Was the work affected by simultaneous operations?
- Could the task only be completed by breaking a procedure or rule?
- Was scheduling of the task involved contrary to that contained in a work management and tracking system?
- Was there sufficient information in the work order to carry out the task?
- Was there an error in the sequence of work orders?
- Was an isolation undertaken on the wrong component?
- Was the job brief by the supervisor adequate?
- Were expected hazards communicated to contractor teams prior to starting work?

Organization

- Are non-conformances reported to management and corrective actions implemented and tracked through to completion by management?
- What is the leaders' level of interest in formal task assignment?
- How is supervisory resourcing decided?
- Does the leader think following the rules or doing the right thing is more important? Why?
- Who draws the line between what is acceptable and unacceptable behaviour around task planning and assignment?

Drift (procedural and practical)

People

- Have the team done the task in the same way in the past without any negative safety impact?
- Do the team ever customize the activity to the situation? If so, how?
- Are there certain ways those involved determine which way to proceed if they do change the way they do the job?
- How stable are the working conditions?
- Is the work usually routine, or does it require a lot of improvisation?
- How often does the team change the way they work? Rarely? Often?
- Looking back over the years or months the task has been carried out, has the way it is done changed?
- Is the way the task was done the same way for all crews and shifts?
- Have those directly involved always done the task the way they did it on the day?

Environment

- Has the location, condition, congestion or other environmental factors changed over a significant period of time?

Equipment

- Was the equipment part of a critical control for a material or fatal risk?
- Has the equipment changed over the years without adequate management of the changes?

Procedures

- How often are the crews included in the review of procedures they are expected to follow?
- Has the procedure been amended or reviewed lately?
- Was the task performed so infrequently that improvements to the conditions were delayed or accepted as "the way it's done"?

Organization

- What level of your thought goes into the long-term drift and trends about the way tasks are done in the business?

Core competency training and awareness induction

People

- Have the team received training on the job for the work they were doing?
- Were the team competent in the job they were doing?
- What induction process was in place?
- How experienced was the team in the task?
- What skills are needed to carry out the work?
- Was a mistake made because the person was not fully qualified to perform the task?
- Were all those involved aware of safe working requirements for this task?
- Were the people involved adequately trained in hazard/risk identification?
- Was the person required to learn on the job but no mentoring or coaching was given?
- Was training not offered because the task is performed so infrequently that training is considered unnecessary?
- Does a gap analysis exist between the core competencies and the training/competency status of the team members?
- Did a supervisor unknowingly assign the wrong person to a task because they were not aware of missed or inadequate training?

Equipment

- Were there changes to the equipment that were not yet included in the training material?

- Was training material related to a subsequently removed piece of plant/equipment?

Procedures

- Is the detail in the training material for this task the same as in the procedures?
- Have those involved read the procedure? If so, when?
- Were there changes to the procedure that were not yet included in the training material?

Organization

- Were enough qualified employees available, either through staffing levels or schedules?
- Was training not provided but should have been?
- Do core competencies exist for the position?
- Is the training material wrong or does it miss important steps?
- Do complete training matrices exist for the area/department?
- Have competency-based training competency assessments been carried out?
- Is training tracked and records made available so supervisors can assign competent people?
- Are supervisors aware of employee capabilities?

Other cognitive biases and heuristics, including internal decision- and sense-making, intense task focus, What-You-See-Is-All-There-Is, plan continuation, etc.

People

- Has there been a spate of incidents similar to the one of interest in the investigation? And has that resulted in a tendency to overestimate the likelihood of an incident related to a different step in the task? I.e. electrical versus fall from height likelihood? (Availability bias)
- Have those creating the risk assessment got to the point of saying "we have finished" too early in the process? This results in an incomplete assessment of the risks of a task. (Completeness bias)
- In reviewing the THA, is there a misalignment between risk and control due to a selective focus by the work team on data and evidence that support their belief of a situation at the time, at the expense of data and evidence that do not support their belief or view? (Confirmation bias)

- Were the work team blind to any subtle cues and changes that went during the development of the incident? (Escalation bias)
- Is there an element of: "I've done this task a thousand times and nothing has ever happened before. I don't understand why it went so wrong this time"? (Gambler's Fallacy)
- Have those involved in the incident adjusted their behaviour in a way that counteracts the intent of the safety device installed? (Peltzman Effect (risk compensation))
- What did people see, or notice, going on around them at the time of the incident?
- Did the way the team saw the incident unfold make sense at the time?
- What was going on in the minds of those involved at the time of the incident?
- How were those involved making sense of their surroundings?
- How much attention was needed to keep on the task when it was being carried out?
- What decisions were made during the event (or when creating the THA) that made sense at the time, but don't seem so clear now?
- What was going on around the area at the time of the incident?
- How much attention did those involved feel they needed to have on the task they were doing?
- What were the team focussing on at the exact time of the incident?
- How often does the way the work is done change? Rarely? Often?
- When the task was assigned, what did the supervisor do to make sure the team understood the details of the task?
- When the task was assigned, what conversations did the supervisor have with the team?
- What were the words the supervisor used to assign the task?
- Did the team imagine that the outcome, as we know it now, was possible?
- What did those involved think would happen when they undertook the task which led to the event?
- How confident were the team that they would succeed in the task?
- Do the team know of any previous incidents or near misses involving this task or similar tasks?
- If so, what was it about that previous experience which seemed relevant?
- Did the task require so much attention that other things were not seen?
- How did the team decide to do the job the way they did?
- What changes were seen as the task progressed?
- Were those involved bored or distracted?
- What is the result of any assessment of personality, safety attitude, motivation, conflict, stress, external influences, i.e. social and domestic pressures?

Efficiency–Thoroughness Trade-Off

People

- If the team had all the time to do the task and had all the tools they needed, in what way would the task look different?
- Do the procedures and other systems drive towards efficiency or thoroughness in getting the tasks done?
- Has any procedural or practical drift resulted in a shift to or away from efficiency or thoroughness over time?

Environment

- Was the task performed so infrequently that improvements to the conditions were delayed or accepted as "the way it's done"?
- Were environmental conditions so extreme that housekeeping routines could not keep up/took inordinate amounts of time?

Organization

- Where do the leaders feel the balance lies with Efficiency–Thoroughness Trade-Off in investigations?
- Where do the leaders feel the balance lies with Efficiency–Thoroughness Trade-Off in safety?

Functional aspects (from the FRAM)

Equipment, environment and organization

- What systems are in play in the incident?
- What are the inputs, outputs, preconditions, resources, controls and time constraints on the functions involved in the incident?
- What was the variation within each of the FRAM aspects (inputs, outputs, preconditions, resources, controls and time)?

Equipment, tools and plant design

People

- Was the task repetitive and subject to ergonomic fatigue?

Environment

- Should the area have been barricaded/protected, but wasn't?
- Were the parts used in the equipment adequate for the operating environment (e.g. non-galvanized steel in wet/corrosive environments)?
- Were displays or alarms placed so that reading them was easy?
- Are emergency controls such as valves able to be operated by anyone regardless of physical stature or strength?
- Was the equipment or work area adequately barricaded to prevent people from entering?
- Did accessing the area expose an individual to hazards not directly related to their task?
- Did the physical environment make it difficult to follow the procedure?
- Did the way the workplace is set out contribute to or hinder safe work?

Equipment

- Did a fault or omission in the original design contribute to the failure?
- Did the preventative maintenance fail to detect a fault?
- Was a control (valve, alarm, etc.) able to be operated by accident (e.g. by bumping into it)?
- Were displays, controls or equipment poorly placed so that using them was a contributing factor?
- Was access/egress to the work area blocked by equipment?
- Did minor differences between two otherwise identical operating systems or control layouts contribute to an error?
- What tools and equipment are normally used to get this task done?
- Were all the tools you would have liked to use easily available?
- Was a scheduled preventative maintenance delayed or ignored?
- Was fall-protection equipment needed but for some reason not used?
- Did workers use inappropriate fall-protection devices?

Procedures

- Was equipment/software/code designed to specifications or standards?
- Should there be a 'safety in design' procedure but one does not exist?

Organization

- Was there a preventative maintenance schedule in place?
- Was protection inadequate for the work?

Culture

People

- Are non-conformances reported to management and corrective actions implemented and tracked through to completion by management?
- What is the leaders' level of interest in safety and investigations?
- Does the leader think following the rules or doing the right thing is more important? Why?
- Who draws the line between what is acceptable and unacceptable behaviour here?
- What is the leaders' reaction to incidents?

Organization

- How is investigation team resourcing decided?
- How does the business learn from other safety events within the company at other locations?
- How does the business learn from other non-company safety events (e.g. Texas City, Macondo, Challenger)?
- Was a corrective action review process in place?
- If not, was corrective action that could have prevented the incident not implemented or not implemented in time?
- What is the process for ensuring the quality of investigations?
- Does the incident investigation process drive minimization of repeat incidents?

Appendix B
Incident Cause Analysis Method process

The ICAM model

If you are planning to act as a facilitator for an ICAM, I strongly suggest that you first make sure you either get some training or make sure your existing skills set is up to date. Reading and studying this book will of course greatly help, but you do need some hands-on training and practice to become effective in facilitating the ICAM process.

As a facilitator, you need to be able to explain the ICAM model to others (Figure B.1). You also need to be able to answer questions about it. This is especially important at the start of an investigation so that the incident investigation team are able to contextualize what the team is try-ing to achieve in the investigation. Below is a description of the ICAM model that I would use in a workshop setting. There is no need for the other members of the investigation team to have a detailed understand-ing of the ICAM model but it is essential that the ICAM facilitator does.

The ICAM model: an explanation

ICAM stands for Incident Cause Analysis Method. It is based on the work of James Reason, a professor of psychology at the University of Manchester in the United Kingdom. Reason did a lot of work on under-standing human error. And the ICAM model is based on his 'Swiss Cheese, Defences in Depth' model of incident causation. It was created for BHP, later BHP Billiton, and is used extensively in many industries across many countries and languages.

In a nutshell, ICAM describes the absent/failed defences, individual/ team actions, task/environmental conditions and organizational factors that contributed to the incident.

- Absent/failed defences are those last-minute defences that were missing or did not work as planned.

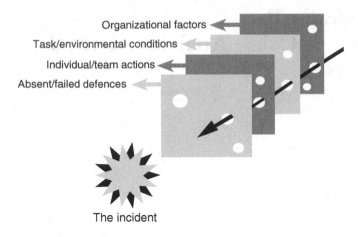

The incident

Figure B.1 ICAM model

- Individual/team actions describe actions that someone did or did not do that led to the incident.
- Task/environmental conditions describe those things that promoted or encouraged the individual/team actions.
- Organizational factors talk to the system-wide issues that created the task/environmental conditions.

I always explain the model by looking at the **individual/team action** slice of the cheese first because this represents Reason's concept of human error, upon which the model is based and is, in many ways, the centre, or core of the ICAM model.

This slice of cheese represents the actions that were taken by either individuals or teams just prior to the incident. The term 'human error' is a label commonly placed on an action only after something has gone wrong. It has a connotation of failure in an individual. People often say that an error was committed, which to me sounds too much like saying that a crime was committed. The latest thinking and science on human factors suggests that the concept of 'human error' has no basis in science, but is, rather unfortunately, an easy category of behaviour. Sidney Dekker talks about this a lot in *Safety Differently* and also in *The Field Guide to Understanding 'Human Error'*. I expect it will unfortunately remain in common use for a while yet.

Keeping that in mind, to me, it is better to think of individual/team actions as actions that people did (or did not) do that resulted in an unexpected outcome. It could be an action that does not align with what the procedure or rule requires. It could also be the omission of an integral step that is required for the task to be completed.

The word 'action' here is important. In order to qualify as an individual/team action, an action must be observable. It cannot be a thought or a decision. It must be something someone did or did not do. It could be someone not filling out a required form (it is theoretically possible to take video footage of them setting up the task but not filling in the form), or it could be an instruction given by a supervisor (you may have heard and it is possible to record the conversation).

As we all know, we make mistakes every day of our lives. We forget where we leave the keys, forget to feed the fish, or we go to the shop without the shopping list or any money.

Even though I describe individual/team actions first in my description of the ICAM model, our first job in an ICAM is to establish which defences were missing or did not work as intended. These are called **absent/failed defences**.

We need to provide these defences to ensure that people are not hurt at work as a result of a mistake or a slip-up. Examples could be ABS or traction control in a vehicle to help avoid an accident. Seat belts, airbags and roll-over protection are other examples of protection, of defences. As you can see from this motor vehicle example, defences can either be designed to prevent an incident from occurring or for minimizing the consequence of an incident after it has happened. After all, a seat belt cannot stop you from having a car accident.

To identify the absent/failed defences, we ask questions such as:

• What could or should have been in place to prevent this incident from happening, but was not in place?
• What was in place to prevent this incident from happening, but did not work as intended or expected?
• What could or should have been in place to minimize the consequences of this incident, but was not in place?
• What was in place to minimize the consequences of this incident, but did not work as intended or expected?

Following the creation of a short list of the absent/failed defences, we establish our list of individual/team actions as described above.

One of the great ideas that Reason helps us with is to understand that there are factors that contribute to us making mistakes, slip-ups and lapses. Many things at work encourage us to not follow the procedures and systems already in place, or to do things in a way that we know was not the best we could have done. In the ICAM, these are described in a cluster called **task/environmental conditions**.

These can range from ineffective task allocation and planning for things like the weather and what personal protective equipment we are provided with, through to poor communication or using procedures that are too detailed and confusing or simply not able to be followed. Such lapses set our people up to fail in their tasks. Giving them the wrong tools, telling them to hurry up or giving mixed messages about what to do – these all increase the likelihood that mistakes will be made and procedures not followed.

So we should ask things like: "What is it about the task or the environment in which we asked people to work that has promoted or encouraged this action to occur?" along with questions derived from Appendix A.

After identifying all of the task/environmental conditions we need to contemplate where they came from. Who created those task/environmental conditions that encouraged people to make poor decisions and carry out erroneous actions? Where did they come from? The answer of course is 'The organization'. The organization could be a department, an operation or the business itself. The organization created the rules that tell us how to write the procedures. The organization tells us how we should purchase things and how we should supply tools and equipment, how to create checklists, how training is done and who should be competent in what skill. It also tells us how to complete risk assessments and assess the impact of changes in the workplace. It is these systems that have produced task/environmental conditions that in turn encourage people to take actions (that we used to call errors or violations) that could have resulted in a severe injury due to the absence of good, solid defences.

To identify these **organizational factors**, we need to look at each task/environmental condition and ask ourselves:

• Where did we go wrong as an organization?
• Where did our systems fail?
• How did we manage to set up a work environment or task that encouraged or promoted the actions that led to the incident?

The answers to these questions let us come up with the organizational factors for the ICAM.

At this point it is very important to ensure that we have the right people in the ICAM team. **Organizational factors** are often strategic and relatively high level, and so the discussion needs to be able to be held at that level. Generally people at a manager level think at a strategic or business-wide level and so having one of them in the ICAM tends to give you better-quality organizational factors. This is one of the reasons why I believe that you should have a manager-level person as the incident investigation leader for detailed incident investigations. I recently reviewed over 400 ICAM reports and found that over 80% of what was declared as organizational factors were in fact task/environmental conditions. This is in part due to the fact that there was not a manager-level person in the investigation team. After building the organizational factors, we then simply create corrective actions for each of the organizational factors and for the absent/failed defences. At this point our ICAM is pretty much all done.

To recap:

Absent/failed defences: the last-minute measures that were designed to prevent the incident, or minimize the consequences, but were either missing or did not work as intended.

Individual/team actions: the actions taken, or not taken, by individuals or teams of people that led to the event.

Task/environmental conditions: the things which were present prior to the event and which promoted or encouraged the individual/team action.

Organizational factors: the high-level systems and processes, leadership and culture aspects that created the task/environmental conditions.

In terms of how we build the ICAM, the absent/failed defences and the individual/team actions are brainstorm-style activities where the facilitator encourages the team to look back through their notes (from the interviews and other data that have been collected along with the timeline and the Hows & Whys activity) to develop the absent/failed defences and then the individual/team actions. I find it beneficial to have the definitions (check questions) of what you are focussing on up on a projector screen as you do this, which will remind the team what you are looking for. We call this the check question, because you should check the language matches once you have decided what to write in each of the sections of absent/failed defences, individual/team actions, task/environmental conditions and organizational factors.

After you have identified the absent/failed defences and the individual/team actions, and they are recorded on large butcher paper up on a wall, fold the butcher paper up so that you can only see the first individual/team action and ask the investigation team: "What is it about the task or the environmental conditions that contributed to or encouraged this action?" From this (looking at each individual/team action in turn), build the task/environmental conditions.

Keep referring to the check question. Repeat the build process for the organizational factors. By this I mean, turn the butcher paper up so that you can only see the first task/environmental condition and then ask the organizational factors questions:

• Where did we go wrong as an organization?
• Where did our systems fail?
• How did we manage to set up a work environment or task that encouraged or promoted the actions that led to the incident?
• What system-wide issues created, or helped create, the task/environmental conditions?

I mentioned this earlier, but it is worth repeating: it is often at this point that we really need to ensure that we have the right people in the ICAM team. We need to ensure the right level people are involved in the discussions around organizational factors at this time. To give you a sense of what the elements of an ICAM look and feel like, here are some examples.

Absent/failed defences

• There was a section of the scaffold without knee or hand rails.
• There was no warning of missing rails or an unsafe condition on the scaff tag.

Individual/team actions

• The operator left the confines of the scaffold to access the valve without using any fall protection.
• The team (operator and supervisor) did not complete a THA prior to the task being undertaken.
• The supervisor instructed the operator to actuate the valve without ensuring the operator had the required competencies, an understanding of the hazards associated with the task or an understanding of the required hazard controls.

Task/environmental conditions

• The operator had not completed any work at height training or awareness sessions.
• The operator understood the instruction given by the supervisor was to do exactly what he did.

• The supervisor was not aware of the requirement to do a THA for all potentially hazardous non-routine tasks and believed that a THA was required only if the "Stop and Think" required it.

Organizational factors

• The Training Needs Analysis process at the operation does not cover basic working at height awareness for operators that are not expected to work at height.
• The operation has not yet implemented the Safe Task Management Standard.
• The process for writing procedures at the operation requires input from those intended to use the procedure but not their approval of the final versions.

Once you have built your list of organizational factors, it is simply a matter of then creating SMARTS actions for each of the organizational factors and the absent/failed defences.

After the ICAM is complete, all the hard work has been done and the draft report has been typed up, it is time for the ICAM leader and the ICAM facilitator to review the draft.

Below is a checklist to help you do that. Answer each question completely, one at a time, before moving on. If you have been asked to review an ICAM, the intention is to provide feedback. Providing feedback is a skill all on its own – and outside the parameters of this book – but I do advise you to get good at it. I find it useful to have the checklist with me during the ICAM. Even though I created the checklist about ten years ago and even though I have reviewed thousands of ICAM reports over those years, when I review an ICAM, I still have the checklist in front of me. The way I do it is to write the numbers 1 to 11 down the side of the first page of the ICAM report and capture as many of my thoughts and comments on the report itself as I review it. This makes it many times easier to provide the feedback especially if you are reviewing a few ICAM reports at the same time. I also encourage facilitators to have the checklist with them as they facilitate an ICAM. It acts as a checklist as you are creating the ICAM just as effectively as when you are reviewing an ICAM report later.

1. Does the timeline include Work-As-Done, Work-As-Normal and Work-As-Intended?
2. Do the Hows & Whys come from the gaps identified between Work-As-Done, Work-As-Normal and Work-As-Intended?

3. ICAM chart: do the contributing factors listed in the ICAM chart (or list) align with the headings?
   - *Absent/failed defences* – last-minute defences that were missing or did not work as planned.
   - *Individual/team actions* – describes actions that someone did or did not do that led to the incident.
   - *Task/environmental conditions* – describes what promoted or encouraged the individual/team actions.
   - *Organizational factors* – describes a system-wide issue that created the task/environmental conditions.
4. Look at each of the individual/team actions and see if there is at least one task/environmental condition that would encourage or promote it as an action.
5. Look at each of the task/environmental conditions and see if there is at least one organizational factor that explains it.
6. Does the Incident Pathway Statement (or ICAM chart/list) clearly tell the story from the organizational factors that produced task/environmental conditions that encouraged or promoted the individual/team actions, in the absence or failure of a defence that led to the event?
7. Do the key learnings come from the investigation and do they summarize what would be useful to others?
8. Do the actions address ALL of the organizational factors and absent/failed defences?
9. Do the actions have SMARTS?
   - Specific
   - Measurable
   - Achievable
   - Relevant
   - Time-bound
   - Sustainable
10. If the actions were in place before the incident, would it have occurred?
11. Are the actions sustainable and will they still be in place and effective in twelve months' time?

If you are asked to provide feedback on a draft ICAM/investigation report, try to remain positive when you are giving the feedback. I recommend you never send your comments as scribbled notes all over someone's ICAM report. And always give feedback face to face, over a video link or at least over the phone. Generally, feedback is and will be taken very personally. Face to face allows you to engage with the person and set them at ease as to the purpose of the feedback – which is, of course, to help them see what you see, or to check that our interpretations are exactly what they meant when they wrote the words. In other words: to help them improve. It is even better to provide feedback throughout the process. Think about sharing your work as it is in the developing stages and asking a peer to provide feedback as you go.

Bibliography

Florence Allard-Poesi:
The Paradox of Sensemaking in Organizational Analysis. Organization 19(2) 2005
Daved Barry and Stefan Meisiek:
Seeing More and Seeing Differently: Sensemaking, Mindfulness, and the Workarts. Organizational Studies 31(12) 2010
Corinne Bieder and Mathilde Bourrier:
Trapping Safety into Rules: How Desirable or Avoidable Is Proceduralization? Ashgate 2013
Erik Brynjolfsson and Andrew McAfee:
The Second Machine Age: Work, Practices, and Prosperity in a Time of Brilliant Technologies. W.W. Norton & Company 2014
Christopher Chabris and Daniel Simons: The Invisible Gorilla: And Other Ways Our Intuition Deceives Us. Harper Collins 2010
W. Chan Kim and Renee W. Mauborgne:
Blue Ocean Strategy: How to Create Uncontested Market Space and Make the Competition Irrelevant. Harvard Business Review Press 2004
Columbia Accident Investigation Board:
Report Volume 1, NASA and the Government Printing Office of the USA 2003 (Obtained from www.nasa.gov/columbia/home/CAIB_Vol1.html)
Todd Conklin:
Pre-Accident Investigations: An introduction to Organizational Safety. Ashgate 2012
Better Questions: An Applied Approach to Operational Learning. CRC Press 2016
Sidney Dekker:
Behind Human Error. 2nd ed. (with David D. Woods, Richard Cook, Leile Johannsen and Nadne Sarter). Ashgate 2010
Drift into Failure: From Hunting Broken Components to Understanding Complex Systems. Ashgate 2011
Patient Safety: A Human Factors Approach. CRC Press 2011
Just Culture: Balancing Safety and Accountability. Ashgate 2012
The Field Guide to Understanding 'Human Error'. 3rd ed. Ashgate 2014

Safety Differently: Human Factors for a New Era. 2nd ed. Ashgate 2015
Sidney Dekker, Erik Hollnagel, David Woods and Richard Cook:
Resilience Engineering: New Directions for Measuring and Maintaining Safety in Complex Systems, Final Report December 2008
Myles Downey:
Effective Coaching: Lessons from the Coach's Coach. 3rd ed. Cengage 2003
Dylan Evans:
Risk Intelligence: How to Live with Uncertainty. Atlantic Books 2012
Bill George:
Discover Your True North: Becoming an Authentic Leader. Wiley 2015
Rob Goffee and Gareth Jones:
Why Should Anyone Be Led by You? What It Takes to Be an Authentic Leader. Harvard Business School Press 2006
Erik Hollnagel:
The ETTO Principle – Efficiency–Thoroughness Trade-Off: Why Things that Go Right Sometimes Go Wrong. Ashgate 2009
FRAM – the Functional Resonance Analysis Method: Modelling Complex Socio-Technical Systems. Ashgate 2012
Safety I and Safety II: The Past and Future of Safety Management. Ashgate 2014
Daniel Kahneman:
Thinking, Fast and Slow. Allen Lane (Penguin) 2011
Max Landsberg:
The Tao of Coaching: Boost Your Effectiveness at Work by Inspiring and Developing Those around You. Profile Books 2003
Mastering Coaching: Practical Insights for Developing High Performance. Profile Books 2015
Robert Long:
Real Risk: Human Discerning and Risk. Scotoma Press 2014
Sally Maitlis and Marlys Christianson:
Sensemaking in Organizations: Taking Stock and Moving Forward. Academy of Management Annals 8(1) 2014
L. David Marquet:
Turn the Ship Around: A True Story of Turning Followers into Leaders. Penguin Random House 2013
James Reason:
Human Error. Cambridge University Press 1990
Managing the Risks of Organizational Accidents. Ashgate 1997
The Human Contribution. Ashgate 2008
A Life in Error: From Little Slips to Big Disasters. Ashgate 2013
Simon Sinek:
Start with Why: How Great Leaders Inspire Everyone to Take Action. Penguin 2011
Paul Slovic:
The Feeling of Risk: New Perspectives on Risk Perception. Routledge 2010

Scott A. Snook:
Friendly Fire: The Accidental Shootdown of US Black Hawks over Northern Iraq. Princeton University Press 2000

Karl E. Weick, Kathleen M. Sutcliffe and David Obstfeld:
Organizing for High Reliability: Processes of Collective Mindfulness. Research in Organizational Behavior 1 1999

John Whitmore:
Coaching for Performance: GROWing human potential and Purpose. Nicholas Brealey 2009

Index

Printed in the United States
by Baker & Taylor Publisher Services